PATTERNS OF RELATING

PATTERNS OF RELATING

An Adult Attachment Perspective

Malcolm L. West
Adrienne E. Sheldon-Keller

Foreword by ROBERT S. WEISS

THE GUILFORD PRESS
New York   London

©1994 The Guilford Press
A Division of Guilford Publications, Inc.
72 Spring Street, New York, NY 10012

Printed in the United States of America

This book is printed on acid-free paper.

Last digit is print number: 9 8 7 6 5 4 3 2 1

Library of Congress Cataloging-in-Publication Data
West, Malcolm L.
    Patterns of relating : an adult attachment perspective /
Malcolm L. West, Adrienne E. Sheldon-Keller.
        p.   cm.
    Includes bibliographical references and index.
    ISBN 0-89862-671-4
    1. Attachment behavior.   2. Adulthood—Psychological
aspects.   I. Sheldon-Keller, Adrienne E.   II. Title.
    BF575.A86W47   1994
    155.6—dc20   93-48128
                                                              CIP

FOREWORD

Attachment theory is not a general theory of relationships. It is, rather, a theory specific to those relationships most important to our feelings of security—relationships on which, as West and Sheldon-Keller note, our feelings of security depend. For children, these are relationships with parents. For adults, they are, foremost, relationships of emotional partnership, of courtship and cohabitation and marriage: relationships whose formation engages the full energies of participants, whose existence provides each of the participants with a sense of anchoring and augmentation, and whose loss gives rise to grief. They are relationships in which the other person is irreplaceable, relationships which permit no substitutes.

Attachment theory has little to tell us about work relationships, friendships, neighboring relationships, and other relationships of community. Indeed, West and Sheldon-Keller demonstrate that these relationships of community are experienced as intrinsically different from relationships of attachment. It is, for example, consistent with work relationships that the departure into retirement of a coworker of many years produces only the briefest experience of distress. Not so the loss from one's life of an attachment figure.

There have been attempts to explain the relationships with which attachment theory deals in simplistic terms of cost and benefit: to view marriage, for example, as a relationship of exchange in which each partner relinquishes some freedom, and accepts some obligations, in order to gain the assured services of the partner. But the phenomena of attachment defy such easy, common sense explanations. Rather, they seem to result from something mysterious and powerful, something indifferent to cool calculation. There is a quality of emotions having taken possession of the person in many of the expressions of attachment: in romantic love and in jealously, in the confusion that regularly accompanies marital separation and the intense grief that regularly accompanies bereavement, and in the desperate anxiety of loneliness. It is adult attachment theory, more than any other theoretical approach, that makes possible the understanding of these phenomena.

Adult attachment theory also provides us with explanations for the many ways in which people behave differently, one from another, in close relationships. One of the established ideas of attachment theory, largely the contribution of Mary Ainsworth and her students, is that for reasons of experience and, perhaps, temperament, different children display different anticipations of caretakers. Working with 2-year-olds, Ainsworth elicited these differences by subjecting the 2-year-olds to a series of parental departures and reunions. Some of the children behaved in ways that suggested that the children remained confident that their parents were essentially reliable despite the parents having briefly absented themselves. Some of the children who did not display such persisting confidence displayed instead an anxious effort to ensure the continued presence and responsiveness of their parents. Some of the children, although equally insecure, seemed to adopt a quite different strategy, in which they gave effort to diminishing or repressing their own feelings of need.

These different approaches to dealing with attachment figures are now customarily referred to as attachment styles. Attachment styles have been shown by longitudinal studies to be persistent throughout childhood. Furthermore, clinical work with adults suggests strongly that the attachment styles of childhood continue on into later life. Although a number of factors might contribute to the stability of attachment styles, including stable social environments, most of the explanation seems to be in a persistence in the way in which close relationships are understood. People seem to operate on the basis of persistent "internal working models" of relationships of attachment that include the likely behavior toward them of people to whom they are close, their own likely behavior in close relationships, and the likely course of close relationships. The same anticipations are brought to new relationships that were brought to old ones.

Obviously the concept of an internal working model is a metaphor. West and Sheldon-Keller are the first, to my knowledge, to grapple with the question of the actual mental processes that might constitute the reality beneath the metaphor. Their proposal is that people make sense of attachment situations as they make sense of anything: by using their perceptions and their affective responses to guide their search for meanings. Earlier experience will have established categories and associations that current perceptions and feelings help elicit. Further experience will then serve to maintain these categories and associations or, alternatively, weaken them in favor of others more consistent with new perceptions and feelings.

This is a formulation that is not only plausible, but almost immediately applicable to the tasks of diagnosis and therapy. As the authors point out, the syndrome descriptions in the American Psychiatric Association's *Diagnostic and Statistical Manual of Mental Disorders* (DSM) are without implication for treatment. The manual, which is used by American therapists who are required by insurance firms to use its classifications, is stubbornly phenomenological. West and Sheldon-Keller are surely right when they hold that in the area of attachment pathologies another approach to classification, based in attachment theory, is preferable just because it is supported by understanding and provides direction for treatment.

If what is wrong with a patient is the persistence of maladaptive attachment strategies, then what has to be achieved with the patient is the replacement of the maladaptive strategies by strategies more likely to lead to satisfactory relationships. The authors propose that for the past to loosen its grip there must be mourning: mourning for the past that had once actually existed and that had been internalized; and mourning for the fantasy, tenacious despite its obvious impossibility, of undoing that past, and magically replacing it with what it should have been. The tasks of mourning include both accepting the past for what it was and recognizing and relinquishing the fantasy that it can be made different.

Even as the patient works toward accepting the past, and so becoming more nearly free of it, West and Sheldon-Keller would have the therapist provide the patient with new anticipations of self, of others, and of relationships of attachment. They would do this through the behavior of the therapist, who by his or her own reliable responsiveness demonstrates that reliable responsiveness is possible. They would do it also through having the therapist encourage the patient to risk acting differently in the world outside the therapist's office, so as to explore the possibility that such relationships can develop differently than the patient anticipates. And they would have the therapist deal directly with the categories of thought elicited in the patient by the patient's experiences, questioning them when appropriate, and offering as alternatives the therapist's own appraisals.

This is a large program for therapy, but how clear is it, and how sensible are its methods and its aims. It is a program, too, that should have wide applicability. While there are disturbances of emotional and cognitive functioning for which quite different therapeutic approaches may be more valuable — one thinks of the phobias for which desensitization procedures might be a therapy of choice, or the depressions that seem so responsive to the right medication — difficulties in relationships of attachment are unquestionably a leading reason for seeking therapeutic help.

An attractive, although perhaps secondary, aspect of West and Sheldon-Keller's approach to therapy is that it will facilitate the evaluation of the success of therapy. All that would be needed to assess therapy's success would be a method for the objective assessment of problems of attachment on entering into therapy and again on departing from therapy. West and Sheldon-Keller have embarked on the task of developing such objective assessments. In the last section of the book, they describe their research in progress on methods of measurement of attachment problems. It is most unusual for a team so perceptive clinically to be so comfortable with the statistical rigors of test construction; but where the same team is able to do both kinds of work, as West and Sheldon-Keller clearly can, their efforts in each enterprise are enriched.

This book is testimony to the maturing field of study of adult attachment, as well as to the field's importance. The author's exemplify what is characteristic of the best current work in this field: serious scholarly concern for building our understanding of adult life together with compassionate awareness of its vicissitudes. To this they have added something new and valuable: efforts to help that are informed and disciplined by adult attachment theory.

ROBERT S. WEISS
Work and Family Research Institute
University of Massachusetts

ACKNOWLEDGMENTS

We are grateful to a number of editors for permission to reproduce articles that appeared first in their journals:

1. The case examples in Chapter 2 appeared in the *Canadian Journal of Psychiatry* (Livesley & West, 1987; West, Sheldon, & Reiffer, 1989) and the *American Journal of Psychotherapy* (West & Keller, 1991).
2. The sections on Avoidant Personality Disorder and Borderline Personality Disorder in Chapter 8 appeared in the *Canadian Journal of Psychiatry* (Sheldon & West, 1990; West, Keller, Links, & Patrick, 1993).
3. The section on Attachment and Affiliation in Chapter 10 appeared in the *British Journal of Psychiatry* (Sheldon & West, 1989).

We are especially grateful to our friend and colleague Sarah Rose who conducted the statistical analyses for Chapter 7. We thank Ronald Aldous for his willingness to discuss the subjects of psychotherapy in ways that have been most helpful to us. Gwyn Nursall prepared the artwork for the pictures in Chapter 7. Our thanks also go to Sharon Panulla and Susan Marples at The Guilford Press for their patience and encouragement.

Finally, we wish to thank Riva West for her editorial assistance during the late stages of manuscript preparation.

CONTENTS

Contents

INTRODUCTION

At its inception in the middle decades of this century, John Bowlby's attachment theory was greeted with resistance and skepticism. Forty years later, attachment concepts are solidly embedded in developmental psychology. It is difficult to imagine the study of child development without reference to Bowlby's vocabulary of secure base, separation and loss, felt security, and exploration. Although in his three volumes on attachment (1969/1982, 1973, 1980) Bowlby elaborated an extremely sophisticated schemata for understanding the psychological consequences of variations in the formation and maintenance of infant–caregiver bonds, the underlying concept of attachment is quite straightforward.

To survive, a human infant must be taken care of. The infant does not exist in an amorphous, undifferentiated world but rather in a world that is centered around a particular "responder" whose actions complement the care-seeking behaviors of the infant. These care-seeking behaviors are called "attachment behaviors." The interactions that result from these behaviors are described as the intermeshing of the infant's attachment system and the adult's care-giving system. Between infant and caregiver, the process of receiving and providing care requires repeated interactions which, viewed as a whole, create a relationship.

But, as Guntrip (1969) has said, each of us lives in two worlds simultaneously, the internal one and the external one. So these care-based interactions have both an internal reality and an external reality for each participant. The internal reality of

1

these interactions creates a superordinate structure, a relationship called "an attachment bond." In the developing internal world of the infant, the attachment bond becomes more than the sum of attachment/care-giving interactions; the attachment bond accrues and includes expectations, emotions, and action patterns. Concurrently, the external and internal worlds of the infant become more extensive, more complex, and more richly textured with emotion.

Just as the interactions for each participant are both internal and external, so their attachment bond is both universal and unique. There is, of course, no universal attachment bond to be found in the external world. But each unique bond between a particular infant and a particular caregiver has familiar elements: elements observed in other attachment bonds between other pairs, although the elements may be expressed very differently. So we observe, quite casually, that one mother picks up her crying baby immediately and another mother deliberately refrains from picking up her baby immediately. Both are responding to the baby's cry, although the responses are expressed in opposite actions.

These observations became the basis for two broad concepts: The attachment bond is universal, at least within our species; and a multiplicity of expressions of the attachment bond are evident. These concepts, in turn, provided the basis for two hypotheses of attachment theory: All humans are influenced by their attachment bonds, and whether this influence is for good or ill depends on the quality of the attachment bond within a particular relationship.

From these theoretical beginnings, researchers in child development got down to the serious business of studying differences in the quality of the attachment bond by empirical means. Methodological access to important aspects of infant–mother bonds was provided by the Strange Situation Protocol (Ainsworth, Blehar, Waters, & Wall, 1978), typified by Karen (1990) as a "Rosetta stone" for developmental psychology. Evidence obtained from Ainsworth's methodology became the basis for the development of a typology of attachment relationships. This typology is both reliable (consistent across subjects, researchers, and time) and valid (meaningfully related to observed phenomena and meaningfully differentiated from other concepts).

In Sroufe and Waters's words (1977), attachment has served as a powerful "organizational construct" within psychosocial research on infants and children. Attachment theory has provided this research with the coherency of language and methodology so essential to scientific inquiry.

Meanwhile, researchers concerned with the interpersonal relationships of adults have long struggled to find such an organizational construct. Among sociologists and related social scientists, the concept of a social support system or social support network (Vaux, 1988) has achieved the most prominence, along with the related ideas of a "confidante" relationship (Brown, Bhrolchain, & Harris, 1975) and the rather ambiguous "significant other" relationship (Cramer, 1990). But despite their popularity among social scientists and the general public alike, the concepts related to social support systems have two pronounced failings:

1. They are descriptive only, lacking a theory of origin and a mechanism of development (e.g., Freeman & Sheldon, 1985).
2. The concepts attend only to the external world and cannot easily or successfully be modified to include the internal reality of all humans (Mueller, 1980).

Research efforts have produced a plethora of findings relating social support constructs to each other and to various indices of coping and adjustment (Cohen & Syme, 1985). Replications generally find different relationships among the variety of dependent, independent, confounding, modifying, and control variables studied (Sarason & Sarason, 1985).

Eschewing theory for description, psychiatric clinicians have tried to incorporate experiential descriptions of relationships into diagnostic categories. Unfortunately, description becomes muddled when not guided by theory. Psychiatric researchers and clinicians are themselves the strongest critics of the resulting diagnostic systems, which demonstrate unacceptable overlap among categories and confusion among criteria (Gorton & Akhtar, 1990).

Psychologists are almost invariably strong proponents of a theory-based descriptive system. The problem is that

psychology seems caught in a Kuhnian dilemma among competing, incompatible paradigms (Kuhn, 1970). These paradigms include traditional psychoanalytic theory, object relations theory,
cognitive and learning theories, and more recently information
processing and neural network theories (Draper & Belsky, 1990).

In a light-hearted vein, one might ask, "Can attachment theory save the day?" The answer is most assuredly "No." To the
degree that it is accepted, it will become a component of the social
network for the social scientist (Heard & Lake, 1986), an alternate descriptive system for the psychiatric clinician (Livesley, Jackson, & Schroeder, 1989), and yet another competing paradigm
for the psychologist (Rice, Fitzgerald, & Lapsley, 1990). Nonetheless, the demonstration that attachment bonds are both universal and specific for adults as well as children is a first step toward
conceptualizing attachment as an "organizational construct" capable of lending continuity to research on important adult relationships.

In this book our main purpose is to define and establish attachment as a primary organizational construct for the study of
essential relationships between adults. The first challenge is to
define attachment relationships for adults using criteria that are
congruent with the definition for infants and children, and suffi-
ciently different from the definition of other relationships for
adults. We *can* identify the criteria of an attachment relationship for infants and children. We *can* identify criteria associated
with close personal relationships for adults. Now we need to identify how these two sets of criteria overlap. If the overlap is substantial and if the overlapping criteria occur primarily in one
relationship for an adult, then we may fairly designate that relationship an attachment relationship. Chapter 1 concentrates on
this particular challenge.

Bowlby (1988b) noted that attachment theory's rise to influence has been mainly restricted to the ranks of developmental
psychologists. But the attachment point of view also has immediate clinical implications. The second challenge is to demonstrate
that, as an organizational construct for adult relationships, attachment is *useful.* Chapter 2 illustrates its clinical import through
the consideration of four case studies.

For attachment theorists, the effects of the caregiver's responsiveness upon the child are the chief data or defining substance of personality. In this view, the child and the attachment environment constitute a dynamic configuration in which the whole relationship is greater than the sum of the interactions that are its parts. Bowlby (1969/1982) cogently argued that rather than positing a unitary developmental sequence, we should try to explain development in terms of the principles used to explain biological development. These topics are discussed in Chapter 3.

The process of interaction between the attachment environment — either that of the present or that of the past — and the individual's psychological world is clarified by Bowlby's concept of the "inner working model." This concept calls proper attention to the representational world in which adults live, the world of their attachment experiences, their expectations and attitudes, their fears. Indeed, research is flourishing on the assessment of this representational world involving the individual's cognitions, interpretations, constructions, and the like. Yet this research tends to pay too little attention to the affective component of the representational world. In Chapter 4 we present the view that models of attachment always have affective content and are centered around a pattern of feelings throughout the individual's life.

The discussion of insecure attachment in Chapter 5 makes apparent our belief that such feelings are inevitably associated with the feared loss of the security invested in the attachment relationship. In this view, patterns of insecure attachment develop in order to protect the individual from remembered and anticipated experiences that are connected with painful feelings of sadness and anxiety. Patterns of insecure attachment are organized to avoid the recurrence of an unbearable threat: the loss of the current attachment relationship. In Chapter 6 we continue the consideration of insecure attachment with an examination of defensive processes from an attachment perspective.

Despite the clinical and theoretical relevance of attachment, its systematic study in adults has been hampered by a lack of self-report and interview measures. In Chapter 7 we describe our methodologies for assessing both the underlying dimensions of adult reciprocal attachment and the primary patterns of insecure attachment.

The clinical descriptions in Chapter 2 touch on patterns of

insecure attachment that can provide a clinically useful description of personality disorders. No diagnostic or classification system exists that makes use of their predominant feature—difficult or impoverished interpersonal relationships—to achieve a reliable differentiation among these disorders. In Chapter 8 we discuss the contribution of patterns of insecure attachment to the differential diagnosis of a subset of personality disorders.

The last step toward establishing the saliency of attachment to the clinician is to consider its role in psychotherapeutic processes and goals. Today it is generally agreed that the therapeutic relationship is of major importance to whatever changes are achieved in psychotherapy. The therapist represents an auxiliary secure base that enables individuals to begin to uncover family secrets and to define landmarks in their past attachment experiences. As we discuss in Chapter 9, the principal aim of an attachment-based psychotherapy is to facilitate the mourning of a yearned for—but never fully experienced—tender, loving relationship with the caregiver.

Attachment is often mistakenly subsumed under either general social relationships or pathological dependency models. Chapter 10 gives special focus to the boundaries that mark attachment off from these related concepts. Evidence is presented from several perspectives, including the reinterpretation of previous studies and the results of studies conducted by ourselves, to indicate that attachment in adults must be defined for investigation primarily in terms of *function* (achievement of felt security) rather than in terms of *structure* (specific behaviors or form of relationship or role-defined other).

We have written this book not because the investigation of adult attachment relationships nears completion, for it is as yet a secondary topic within the larger and richer field of infant and childhood attachment. Our hope is that this book will stimulate interest among researchers, clinicians, and students in considering adult attachment not as a derivative from either infant attachment or social support research, but rather as an intriguing, inviting, and rewarding field of study in its own right.

ONE

THE DEFINITION OF ADULT
RECIPROCAL ATTACHMENT

I n *The Ghost in the Machine* (1967), the third book in his trilogy on the nature of creative innovation, Arthur Koestler described the reductionism, built on a mechanistic conception of human life and psychology, that flourished during the first half of this century. As background for the discussion of the development of attachment theory, we propose similarly that the traditional psychoanalytic conception of the child's tie to the mother rested upon three reductionistic "pillars of unwisdom":

1. The young infant is in a state of primary narcissism (or as Margaret Mahler [Mahler, Pine, & Bergman, 1975] was later to call it, a state of infantile autism) in which the infant experiences himself[1] as self-sufficient and consequently has no need for personal relatedness.
2. The object in this young infant's world is not truly a person but rather a vehicle for drive gratification.
3. The object later becomes a person to the young infant through interactions conditioned by feeding.

As Sroufe (1986) indicates, there is a sense in which Bowlby's (1969/1982, 1973, 1980) entire trilogy on attachment is a corrective reproach to the view that relatedness is secondary to the satisfaction of basic drives such as orality. In Volume 1, Bowlby (1969/1982) reveals the primacy of attachment not only in humans but in all altricial animals. While tracing the universality of attachment behavior, he offers a wide range of illustrations of behavioral organization in subhuman species. By the end

7

of Volume 1, the reader can have no doubt that Bowlby's theory is grounded in ethology. But it does not follow that Bowlby is primarily interested in the instinctive nature of behaviors that promote and maintain attachment. Were Volume 1 devoted to a catalogue of instinctive attachment behaviors in infancy, it would have little relevance to later life. Instead, Bowlby's interest is in the systems that control expression of these behaviors.

BEHAVIORAL CONTROL SYSTEMS

The central thesis of attachment theory is that attachment in humans, and in many other species, is a particular type of biologically "wired-in" control system, specifically a *behavioral control system*. Behavioral control systems organize and direct *behaviors* or activities to achieve specific *set goals,* which had survival value within the "environment of evolutionary adaptedness" (Stevenson-Hinde & Hinde, 1990, p. 65). Within any one species animals with better functioning control systems had greater probability of surviving to reproductive age. Consequently, control systems eventually become species-wide.

The set goal of a behavioral control system is defined as:

> either a time-limited event or an on-going condition either of which is brought about by the action of behavioral systems that are structured to take account of discrepancies between instruction and performance. . . . A set-goal is not an object in the environment but is either a specified motor performance . . . or *the achievement of a specified relation* [with] some object in or component of the environment. (Bowlby, 1969/1982, p. 69; emphasis added)

The ability to take account of discrepancies between the set goal and the current condition, and to modify responses accordingly, is an important component of control systems; that is, a control system always includes mechanisms for *feedback*. The operation of the system is therefore referred to as goal-corrected. This type of system is differentiated from a fixed action system, which may be oriented toward a goal, but is not subject to regulation of expression by feedback mechanisms (Hinde, 1975). As we shall see, the set goal of attachment as a behavioral system is defined in terms of a *specified relation* to a particular other.

The concept of a set goal is important to understanding the crucial difference between *cause* and *function* in the context of control systems. "Causes" refer to the stimuli activating control systems; "functions" refer to the purposes of activation. Thus, for example, a rapid drop in ambient temperature can *cause* shivering; the *function* of shivering is to raise body temperature. In particular, the function of a behavioral control system determines the system's contribution to the probability of survival. Expressed behaviors are the means of achieving the system's set goal. The set goal is the means of accomplishing the system's function.

Control systems, as are other abilities of the organism, are subject to developmental change and elaboration (Bowlby, 1969/1982). The conditions for activation, termination, and suppression; the nature of feedback information; and the associated behaviors are each modified as the organism develops. In addition, the integration among behavioral systems generally becomes more elaborate with development. In the earliest stages of life, behavioral systems are usually competitive, with one system at a time predominating. The simplest relational organization is a linked chain wherein termination of one system serves as an activation signal for another system. If an activation signal is shared, the set goals of systems can become integrated.

The most complex organization is a hierarchical structure, such that each component is a behavioral system in its own right, through many levels to an overall system. Koestler (1967) terms such components "holons" and notes that the overall system remains stable as long as the "integrative" and "self- assertive" tendencies of the component holons are in dynamic equilibrium.

One final elaboration is possible; but this elaboration reaches full expression only in humans. This is the modification and control of control systems themselves by higher processes of consciousness and cognition. Bowlby (1969/1982, p. 80) refers to the construction of "working models" that are based on actual experiences but are used to extrapolate those experiences to novel situations. Bowlby postulates that, to be effective, working models must be internally consistent, must include realistic abstractions from the environment and the self (i.e., an awareness of one's own abilities, limitations, and potentials), must be permeable (i.e., subject to revision due to new information), and must, at least at times, be consciously explored.

In summary, a properly functioning behavioral control system responds to causes for activation with a variable pattern of behaviors such that progress toward a set goal is subject to correction through feedback. The set goal confers evolutionary advantages. Signals or causes for activation, termination, and suppression of the control system are often complex and multi-determined. The control system is subject to developmental elaboration, both through increasingly sophisticated connections among systems and through modification by higher processes.

ATTACHMENT AS A BEHAVIORAL CONTROL SYSTEM IN INFANCY

Now that the key components of behavioral control systems in general have been delineated, we can offer a straightforward description of the attachment behavioral system in infancy. The key components, as they apply to the attachment behavioral system in infancy (i.e., from early infancy to about 24–30 months old) are summarized in Table 1.1.

The attachment behavioral system is a control system whose *function* is protecting the altricial animal from danger, specifically, the danger of predation. *More generally, the function of the attachment behavioral system is to ensure safety and security, and thereby to enhance the chances of survival.* This safety is achieved through proximity to the primary caregiver, which is the set goal of the attachment behavioral system. The primary information modifying the behavioral responses to activation (i.e., the primary *feedback* information) is simply the response of the caregiver. Attachment in infancy is not truly integrated with other behavioral systems; instead, it predominates: Activation of the attachment behavioral system will supersede all other behavioral systems (Weiss, 1982). Since the infant has limited cognitive abilities, the modification of the attachment system by higher processes is minimal. The primary causes of activation and termination, and the primary attachment behaviors, are listed in Table 1.1.

TABLE 1.1. Attachment during Infancy

Source:	Behavioral control system
Funtion:	Safety (protection from danger)
Set goal:	Proximity to a specific caregiver
Relationship type:	Complementary
Feedback information:	Response of caregiver
Integration with other systems:	Limited—attachment overwhelms others
Modification by higher processes:	Minimal
Causes of activation:	Distance from primary caregiver
	Condition of child
	Behavior of primary caregiver
	Environmental stressors
Causes of termination:	Vary with intensity of activation:
	High: physical contact with caregiver
	Moderate: sight or sound of caregiver
	Low: proximity to a substitute
Causes of suppression:	Rare
Associated behaviors:	Approach behaviors, for example:
	Reaching
	Clinging
	Following
	Signaling behaviors, for example:
	Crying
	Babbling
	Calling

The point must be emphasized that, in infancy, attachment is a very powerful but very simple behavioral control system.

The relationship between infant and caregiver is described as *complementary* (Hinde, 1976); that is, each partner exhibits distinct behaviors in relation to the other, and although these behaviors are not the same they interlock. The infant's behaviors are consistently care seeking; the parent's behaviors are consistently care giving. Bowlby (1969/1982) has described this process as the intermeshing of two different control systems: the attachment control system of the infant and the care-giving control system of the parent.

Control System versus Affectional Bond

Most definitions of attachment mention or imply that all attachments are affectional bonds. For Bowlby (1977, p. 201), attachment is "the propensity of human beings to make strong affectional bonds to particular others." For Ainsworth et al. (1978, p. 302), attachment is defined as "the affectional bond or tie an infant forms between himself and his mother—a bond that tends to be enduring and independent of specific situations." Concerning the adult, Ainsworth (1989, p. 711) notes "that an 'attachment' is an affectional bond, and hence an attachment figure is never wholly interchangeable with or replaceable by another." The idea of attachment as an affectional bond has not so much modified as supplemented the idea of attachment as a behavioral control system. Sroufe and Waters (1977, p. 1185), for example, make the point that at this stage of our knowledge, Bowlby's "control system model requires elaboration to yield a truly viable developmental construct." For this reason, they emphasize the goal of attachment as "felt security" and focus their attention on attachment as an affective tie rather than as a control system.

Since then, the concept of felt security as the set goal of attachment in periods of development beyond infancy has won wide acceptance. For example, a reading of the recently edited book *Attachment in the Preschool Years* (Greenberg, Cicchetti, & Cummings, 1990) reveals a chapter entitled "Classification of Attachment as a Continuum of Felt Security."

Taking issue with Sroufe and Waters conception, Ainsworth (1990) argues that proximity to the attachment figure *enables* the individual to feel secure. In the same vein, Main (1990) distinguishes two different "conditional behavioral strategies," primary and secondary strategies. The primary system is context-sensitive in that it continually monitors the degree of proximity to the attachment figure.

All this may be illuminated by carefully distinguishing function from set goal. Function answers the question "why." Set goal answers the question "how." As we have seen, the function of a behavioral system is defined as the contribution that system makes to survival. The function of attachment is protection from danger (John Bowlby, personal communication, July 11, 1986). The set goal of a system is the means the organism can use to accomplish the function. The set goal through which the function of attachment is achieved is proximity to an attachment figure. And if one thinks of the maintenance of proximity to an attachment figure at later ages as increasingly an internalized representational process, then one may, as we suggest below, keep it as the set goal of attachment in adults.

Empirical Work

Infant attachment has been the subject of intensive investigation for almost four decades (Watkins, 1987). Consequently, the goals of the research have evolved considerably. Briefly, the investigation of infant attachment can be organized under four goals:

1. Identification of the behaviors associated with activation of the attachment behavioral system (e.g., Ainsworth & Wittig, 1969; Bowlby, 1969/1982; Main, 1977).

2. Organization of the behaviors into discrete patterns reflecting qualitatively different relationships with the caregiver (e.g., Ainsworth et al., 1978; Main & Solomon, 1986; Waters & Deane, 1985).

3. Investigation of the continuity of these patterns into early childhood (e.g., Feldman & Ingham, 1975; Lamb, 1985; Main, Kaplan, & Cassidy, 1985; Greenberg, Cicchetti, & Cummings, 1990).

4. Correlation of attachment patterns with indices of adjustment and psychological well-being (e.g., Cohn, 1990; Matas, Arend, & Sroufe, 1978; Erickson, Sroufe, & Egeland, 1986; Lewis, Feiring, McGuffog, & Jaskir, 1984; Fagot & Kavanagh, 1990).

These goals can be viewed as forming a hierarchical system, with each goal both building on and encompassing previous goals. The system rests on the first goal, the identification of attachment behaviors. All arguments about the differential organization, development, and effects of qualitatively different attachment relationships are inferences from the observation and classification of attachment behaviors.

The most successful and widely used strategy for identifying and classifying attachment behaviors is the Strange Situation Protocol developed by Mary Ainsworth (Ainsworth et al., 1978).

The infant's behaviors in this structured interaction are the data used to define four general patterns of attachment relationships: secure, avoidant, ambivalent, and disorganized (Ainsworth et al., 1978; Main & Solomon, 1986).

The key points are that the assessment of infant attachment relies exclusively on *behaviors,* and that because of the predominance of the attachment behavioral system in infancy, the behaviors are evoked by a very mild stressor (brief separation from the caregiver in a safe environment). Almost all subsequent empirical and theoretical work on attachment in infancy is based on Ainsworth's methodology.

THE ATTACHMENT SYSTEM IN ADULTHOOD

Due in part to the persistent popularity of the phrase "I am very attached to my . . . ," most authors readily assume that attachment persists throughout the life span as a special type of affectional bond. Rutter (1981, p. 274) notes, "It is clear that deep attachments and loving bonds are an important feature of adult life." The subtitle of an oft-cited article by Henderson (1977) is "The Function of Attachment in Adult Life." But there are several problems in proceeding beyond common usage to extrapolate from attachment as it is observed in infants and young children to adults. If attachment as an affectional bond is to play a meaningful role in the differentiation of adult social relationships, then the definition of attachment relationships for adults should fulfill three prerequisites:

1. It should be theoretically congruent with the definition of attachment for children and infants.
2. It should delineate how attachment for adults differs from attachment for infants and children.
3. It should differentiate attachment from other social relationships.

Bowlby's (1977) organization of attachment theory in "The Making and Breaking of Affectional Bonds" includes statements relevant to each prerequisite. Bowlby states that, "Whilst especially evident during early childhood, attachment behavior is held to characterize human beings from the cradle to the grave. . . . There is nothing intrinsically childish or pathological about it" (pp. 129, 131). Bowlby also touches on the differentiation of childhood and adult attachment: While the initial attachment patterns of infancy and childhood develop in direct response to and as a result of the caregiver's actions (or failures to act), the attachment patterns of adults arise largely from working models of the attachment figure and of the self, built on childhood experiences and significantly affecting the adult's ability to form new attachment relationships. Finally, Bowlby refers to " . . . a mass of evidence to support the view that exploratory activity is of great importance in its own right" (p. 133). He goes on to propose that, because exploratory activity leads a person away from his or her secure base with the attachment figure, it is "antithetical" to attachment behavior. According to Bowlby, "In healthy individuals the two kinds of behavior normally alternate" (p. 133). Bowlby's theory of attachment, therefore, encompasses the identified prerequisites for the meaningful definition of attachment in adults.

In a cogent article, Robert Weiss (1982) also elaborates these concepts. Weiss first describes the three central criteria defining an attachment relationship in infancy (p. 172):

1. Proximity-seeking: "The infant will attempt to remain within protective range of the attachment figure."
2. Secure base: "In the presence of an attachment figure, so long as there is no threat, an infant will give indication of comfort and security."
3. Separation protest: "Threat to continued accessibility to the attachment figure or actual separation . . . will give rise to protest and to attempts to ward off the attachment figure's loss or to regain the attachment figure's presence."

Then, based on evidence from interview studies, Weiss states that relationships "that meet the three criteria for attachment are to be found regularly" in adults (1982, p. 172).

Childhood–Adult Differences

Weiss (1982) delineates three characteristics that differentiate attachment in adults from attachment in children (p. 173):

1. In adults, attachment relationships are typically between peers, rather than between care receiver (infant) and caregiver (parent).
2. Attachment in adults is not as liable as attachment in infancy to overwhelm "other behavioral systems.
3. Attachment in adults often includes a sexual relationship.

Mild stressors do not evoke attachment behaviors in the adult because the adult can retain confidence in the availability of the attachment figure in the absence of physical proximity (Hinde & Stevenson-Hinde, 1976); further, the adult has internal (cognitive) strategies as well as external (behavioral) strategies for responding to activation of the attachment system (Blass & Blatt, 1990; Braito, Breci, & Keith, 1990; Main et al., 1985). As Guntrip (1974, p. 830) has said, in another context, as adults we "live in two worlds at once, the inner mental world and the external material world, and constantly confuse the two together." The adult comes to depend heavily on an internal representation of his or her relationship to the attachment figure, a representation begun with an early "working model" (Bowlby, 1969/1982) and elaborated and extended through years of successive and varied attachment experiences. Although Bowlby preferred the term "working model" to emphasize the dynamic nature of the construct, many authors use the terms "working model" and "representational model" interchangeably, or prefer the term "representational model" (Hamilton, 1985; Main et al., 1985; Bretherton, 1985). The term "working model" is used consistently in this work.

While the working model is certainly a higher process modifying expression of the attachment behavioral system, it cannot easily be classified as simply one component of the system. It is better understood as the mechanism mediating development in most components of attachment. One's internal understanding of the relationship between oneself and one's attachment figure influences activation, termination, and suppression of the attachment system; supplants, in many instances, the role of concrete behaviors; provides feedback to the system, and influences the system's sensitivity to other feedback. The pervasiveness of the working model is summarized in Table 1.2.

The working model does not completely supplant attachment behaviors. Especially in times of major life crises, attachment behaviors are frequently both visible and predominant for the adult (e.g., crying, hugging, restlessness when alone, nonresponsiveness to external events). Bowlby (1969/1982, p. 208) warns that to call such behaviors "regressive is indeed to overlook the vital role that [attachment] plays in the life of man."

Differentiation

Weiss (1982) differentiates attachment from other relationships for adults. This differentiation is based largely on the effects of the absence of different types of bonds. In the absence of an at-

TABLE 1.2. Attachment during Adulthood

Source:	Behavioral control system + learned response system
Funtion:	Safety (protection from danger)
Set goal:	Proximity to a specific peer-partner
Relationship type:	Reciprocal
Feedback information:	Working model
	Response of partner
Integration with other systems:	"Holon" within pair-bonding system
Modification by higher processes:	Working model is the source of pervasive modification
Causes of activation:	Working model
	Extended unavailability of partner
	Behavior of partner
	Life crises
Causes of termination:	Working model
	Responsiveness of partner
	Return to environmental homeostasis
Causes of suppression:	Working model
	Learned responses
	Behavior of partner
	Cognitive control
Associated behaviors:	Use of the working model
	Approach behaviors
	Signaling behaviors

tachment bond, Weiss observed, individuals experienced persistent "loneliness" that was not relieved by participation in a friendship network. In contrast, individuals "without access to a community of others" experienced distress associated with isolation. In Weiss's terms: "What they lacked might be characterized as "affiliation"—associations in which shared interests and similarity of circumstances provided a basis for mutual loyalty and a sense of community" (p. 174). This "affiliation" need is thus congruent with both the "psychosocial supplies" (Caplan, 1974) provided by the social network and with the exploratory behavioral system that Bowlby characterized as "antithetical" to the attachment behavioral system. Some theorists (Heard & Lake, 1986; Henderson, 1977) regard phenomena brought under the heading of affiliation as being no different from attachment. Their approach to attachment in adults is to define attachment as a subset, identified by intensity and intimacy, of an individual's social support or affiliative network. This problem of boundaries, or the way in which attachment is delimited and distinguished from other types of social relationships, will be considered in Chapter 10.

Complementarity versus Reciprocity

One final issue remains: the nature of the relationship between the attachment-bonded pair. In infancy and early childhood, we have noted, the relationship is *complementary,* with the infant's care-seeking behaviors complementing the parental care-giving behaviors. A permanent complementary relationship of this type is neither usual nor psychologically healthy for the adult (Gewirtz, 1972). The normal primary relationship for the adult is a *reciprocal* pair-bond with a peer (Weiss, 1974). In reciprocal relationships, one partner is not perceived to be stronger or better able to cope nor are the behaviors distinct between each member of the pair. Each partner has a pair-bond (usually a sexual pairbond) to the other; either partner can exhibit the behaviors characteristic of the bond. But, as Hinde and Stevenson-Hinde (1976) point out, reciprocity can include intermittent interludes of complementarity. The difference of adult attachment from infant attachment is that the complementarity is not always in the same direction. At times one partner may be the caregiver for the other;

at other times the roles can be reversed. (For the sake of clarity, the argument is confined throughout to the prototypical case: In the individual case, the relationship can exhibit these potentials to greater or lesser degrees through a range of normality and including pathological extremes.)

In times of perceived danger when security is threatened, reciprocal relationships can function as complementary relationships. A pair-bonded peer can serve the same role as an attachment-bonded caregiver. From the ethological perspective of survival advantages, bonds to a healthy adult peer should confer greater advantages than bonds to aging parents. Thus, the shift of the set goal of attachment from proximity to a caregiver to proximity to a peer is congruent with the function of attachment.

Definition of Adult Reciprocal Attachment

In concert with the theory and work of Bowlby and Weiss, we restrict the definition of adult attachment to *dyadic relationships in which proximity to a special and preferred other is sought or maintained to achieve a sense of security.* As adults, most of us plan our lives on the basis of an anticipated future with a special other in the expectation of finding security and permanence in an enduring relationship. A qualification is, of course, necessary. The phrase "expectation of finding security" places the emphasis upon the *search for security* and implies that not all attachment relationships *are secure.* Consistent with this qualification, then, we may say that adults seek relational proximity to a particular person (as children do) which, if found, promotes, enhances, or restores security.

BOWLBY AND OBJECT RELATIONS THEORY

Such, then, is the continuity of the function of attachment from infancy to adulthood. Bowlby's book, *Attachment* (1969/1982), propounded new ideas about child development and was a major conceptual landmark on the new path of object relations theory. Inasmuch as Bowlby's training and initial theoretical orientation was within the object relations field of psychoanalysis, we find it appropriate to provide a brief summary of the relationship between attachment theory and object relations theory.

The theories of traditional psychoanalysis (Brenner, 1955; Fenichel, 1945; Freud, 1926) model individual psychological reality as an internal and separate phenomenon, arising from basic drives rooted in physiology, and having content that precedes and determines social experiences. Object relations theorists, in contrast, emphasize the precedence of the *interactional* field, beginning where traditional psychoanalytic theory ends, with interpersonal relationships.

In 1952 Fairbairn argued that if psychoanalysis was to solve the problem of adhesiveness to early object ties, its practitioners would have to move beyond total faith in the pleasure principle. He proposed that loyalty to "bad objects" is independent of the pleasure principle and develops under the impact of object seeking, independent of determinants in the drive system and of conflicts between drives and defenses. Fairbairn argued not only for the primacy of object seeking, but also, like Bowlby, for the idea that the motivation for relatedness is innate.

In his effort to give a biological grounding to object seeking, Bowlby may be said to have put more into the organism from the start than other object relations theorists. For example, Winnicott's (1965) account of the development of a real sense of self is a purely psychological theory in which the infant's self is viewed as formed and sustained by the "facilitating" environment provided by the caregiver. Bowlby's emphasis upon the instinctive nature of attachment behavior, however, does not diminish the importance of the early development of attachment as a result of the interplay between the parental care-giving system and the infant's attachment system.

Bowlby thus represents the infant in terms of complex relatedness capacities and opened the way to the study of relationships as grounded in biology. But in explaining how personality is built up, Bowlby, like Winnicott, focuses largely on the external object as the most important source of influence on the individual. As summarized by Sroufe (1986, p. 845), Bowlby's central hypothesis is that "the quality of any attachment relationship depends on the quality of care experienced with that partner." Fairbairn (1952) also begins with the dyadic unit and the child seeking after objects. If the actual caregivers are "lost" (i.e., emotionally unavailable), and thereby become "bad objects," they are internalized and retained as intrapsychic presences within the child. Although Fairburn regards the developing child as enmeshed in a relational network, he subsequently focuses for the most part on relationships to objects *within* the individual.

An accent on the internal object tends to accompany an accent on earlier rather than later events in explaining the consequences of adverse experiences on normal development. Within object relations theory, normal development is modeled as an invariant sequential and hierarchical process, proceeding through necessary stages. Each stage builds on previous stages; failure at one stage results in cessation of progress. Continuity with the past is accented; adult relationships are modeled as fixed residues of early childhood experiences (Blanck & Blanck, 1974; Mahler et al., 1975; Balint, 1968).

As we discuss in detail in Chapter 3, attachment theory encompasses a different developmental model, as expressed in Waddington's (1967) model of branching pathways. At birth, there are a large number of potential pathways to maturity. Varied experiences progressively narrow these choices and can constrain the choices into maladaptive pathways. Outcome is not "overdetermined" by past experiences but rather "restrained from alternative pathways." Unlike traditional psychoanalytic and object relations theories of development, attachment theory does not define discrete "stages" of development, but rather formulates a theory of developmental continuity, built on the elaboration and expression of the internal working model of attachment.

CONCLUSION

Bowlby (1979) used ethology and evolutionary requirements as the foundation of his theory. In ethology, the work of pioneers such as Lorenz (1952) and Tinbergen (1951) had much the same effect as, in an earlier century, the work of Mendel. The findings that captured the imagination of Bowlby, a renegade psychoanalyst, were that complex and stable behavioral patterns, including behaviors that seemed to have a high affective content, arose from evolutionary necessities. Bowlby came to understand the first affectional bond of a human infant not as the result of a psychological drive, nor as a result of the search for object constancy, but simply as a result of natural selection: in other words, as an important and necessary contribution to survival of the species.

This approach, however, left "man qua man" as the missing link in the theory. At this stage in the development of attachment theory, attachment was conceived as similar to imprinting in precocial animals and would be of interest primarily to ethologists and behaviorists. Attachment theory was "saved" from this narrow application by Bowlby's developmental orientation. In his writings he emphasized the consequences throughout life of common variations in the way a caregiver responds to a child's attachment behaviors. This variability defines the conditions favoring or hampering the development of secure attachment. The accent on attachment as an interactional system, though it had its roots in the theory of attachment propounded by Bowlby, has been mainly supported by Ainsworth's methodology for classifying patterns of infant attachment.

We began by focusing on the continuity between attachment in infancy and attachment in adulthood, and the importance of distinguishing the unique *function* of attachment relationships. If one thinks of attachment as an organization that exhibits some continuity even as it changes throughout the individual's life, then one may use the criteria for infant and child attachment as a frame of reference to describe the features of normal adult attachment. Although no component of attachment remains unchanged from infancy to adulthood, the original formulation of attachment theory not only allows but indeed postulates such revisions. Further — and critically — what does remain unchanged is the *function* of attachment. The function of attachment, the provision of safety and security, remains constant throughout the life span, although the mechanisms of achieving this function change and develop with maturation. Since the original theory is built on a functional argument, a strong case can be made for the relevance and necessity of investigating attachment in all stages of life.

Given that the function of attachment is the maintenance

of safety and security, attachment relationships should be especially crucial in times of life crises and in determining successful adaptation as adults. Bowlby (1988a, p. 8) has stated that "the extent to which [each individual] becomes resilient to stressful life events is determined to a very significant degree by the pattern of attachment he or she develops during the early years." In the remainder of this book we will establish the theoretical and empirical components necessary to investigate, understand, and intervene with patterns of attachment in adulthood.

TWO

THE RELEVANCE OF ADULT
RECIPROCAL ATTACHMENT

mportant as it is that the general principles of attachment theory be established, our theories are only meaningful if they capture the life experiences of real people. The clinical application of attachment theory and research is increasingly a source of interest within the ranks of those who practice counseling and psychotherapy (Dozier, 1990; West, Sheldon, & Reiffer, 1989; Guidano & Liotti, 1983; Jones, 1983; Peterfreund, 1983). Practitioners are drawn to the subject by the expectation that it will give them a better understanding of people for their daily clinical work. In expressing some disappointment that the clinical relevance and usefulness of the attachment perspective has not been fully realized, Bowlby observed (1988b, p. 12):

> whereas attachment theory was formulated by a clinician for use in the diagnosis and treatment of emotionally disturbed patients and families, its usage hitherto has been mainly to promote research in developmental psychology. Whilst I welcome the findings of this research as enormously extending our understanding of personality development and psychopathology, and thus as the greatest clinical relevance, it has none the less been disappointing that clinicians have been so slow to test the theory's uses.

The field of attachment, which rests today on an expansive body of knowledge, has provided general principles of development and a means of specifying the lasting effects of common variations in the way a parent responds to a child's attachment behaviors. When interest is focused upon the *individual*, however, the object of study must also include the *unique outcome* of a set of developmental adjustments. The study of attachment cannot therefore avoid also being a study of the individual case.

Moreover, we take the view that an introduction to the study of attachment can best be accomplished by showing its main themes as they are displayed in actual lives. An outline for presenting the attachment story of a single individual can also be considered an outline for subsequent chapters. The things we would wish to know in order to understand the attachment pathway taken by an individual foreshadows quite nicely the ground to be covered by this book.

One's understanding of a given case needs to go beyond a mere compilation of events in the individual's attachment history. As well, these events cannot be related by mere addition; rather, an attempt must be made to lay hold of the organizing theme among them. In other words, to say that the individual is the sum of his or her attachment experiences is to overlook the coherence of attachment relationships (Sroufe & Fleeson, 1988). Various attachment events in an individual's life are, in this view, both the cause and the consequences of relatively enduring *patterns of relating.*

Four attachment stories are presented here for the purpose of previewing the main topics to be covered later. All of the individuals were seen in long-term individual psychotherapy in the outpatient clinic of a large teaching hospital. The first individual had suffered mixed symptoms of depression and anxiety for the past 10 years. These symptoms approximated the diagnosis of dysthymic disorder from the third revised edition of the *Diagnostic and Statistical Manual of Mental Disorders* (DSM-III-R; American Psychiatric Association, 1987). The second individual's problems were consistent with what would be described clinically as schizoid (Fairbairn, 1952; Guntrip, 1969), as "false self" (Winnicott, 1965), or as avoidant personality-disordered (DSM-III-R). The third and fourth individuals had been diagnosed according to DSM-III-R criteria as suffering from dependent and passive-aggressive personality disorders, respectively. The case studies were chosen to highlight the close connection between personality pathology and patterns of insecure attachment.

FOUR CASE STUDIES

Case Example 1

Mary, a woman in her late 20s, sought therapy upon receiving word two weeks earlier that her mother, who lived in another province, was ill. She felt compelled to have her mother come live with her; this precipitated anxiety and depression. Mary began the first interview feeling depressed and stating, "I've always been afraid." She wondered aloud: "Why can't I be different? Why must this old guilt always come up and make me feel responsible for my mother?" Her relationship with her mother had been discussed with her family doctor who added to his prescription of an antidepressant the admonition that Mary forget about her mother and live her own life. At the conclusion of the first session, the therapist remarked that he had the impression that Mary had long served as an "antidepressant" for her mother. This comment had a remarkable impact upon Mary and became over the course of therapy a touchstone of her relationship to her mother.

Mary was the youngest of two children. Between Mary and her sister, who was 15 years older, there had not been much intimacy. In fact, her sister had left home when Mary was 5. Now, as adults, the relationship between them had grown closer; indeed, Mary had moved to take a secretarial job in a city where her sister lived in order to be able to see her more often.

In therapy, Mary revealed a picture of her mother as fragile, easily upset over trifles, making mountains out of molehills. "She was always unhappy — there was something wrong all the time." Her mother was fearful of people, critical of them — "She never had a kind word for anyone" — and avoided contact with them. During Mary's childhood and early adolescent years, her mother was subject to outbreaks of depression, severe enough on occasion to require hospitalization. At these times, her father had reacted to the crises by withdrawal: "When things went wrong, he got out of the house, walked away." Fatefully, the responsibility for her mother fell to Mary.

An episode recalled from childhood dramatically captures the responsibility Mary felt for her mother's welfare. In this scene, her father sent her into the garden to speak with her mother.

She found her mother running around, pulling her hair out, and screaming "It's my nerves, I can't go on." In recalling other similar incidents, Mary said, "She didn't try to control herself." She feared her mother would take her life or desert her. In response, Mary appeased her mother, catering to her and serving her in many ways in the hope of making her happy. Not surprisingly, given the nature of her mother's threats, Mary had been anxiously attached to her mother. Yet when she was with her she felt "lonely and lost."

Mary reported that she would often sit by the window and look out, feeling uncertain about whether she was loved or not. She remembered her home as empty and pervaded by a deadening glumness. As noted, Mary was bound to her mother by the need to look after her. Her mother had always been possessive. Mary related the many ruses her mother used "to keep me under her thumb." For example, her mother used her suffering to make a claim upon Mary; she made Mary feel indebted by her constant reminder of "all that I have done for you"; and, when Mary was a teenager, her mother made Mary feel delinquent in her attention to her. The result of these machinations was that, because of her mother, Mary always had the feeling that she was suffocating. As she put it, "I couldn't stand it." But then she rhetorically asked, "Why did I keep going back to her? It seems the more unhappy you are, the more you want to go back. I suppose you hope it will be different."

Although Mary had done very well academically and had the ambition to attend university, she received no encouragement from her parents. She enrolled instead in a secretarial course at a local business school. She has been employed for the past 7 years as a secretary. In this position, Mary's strong inner tendency toward deference and an eagerness to take on chores that ought to have been left to others resulted in her assuming responsibilities beyond the duties of her job.

Mary's pattern in her love affairs reflected a continuation of self-surrender. Sexual interest flowed relatively freely to a succession of partners, all of whom were younger than her. Unhappy and insecure, these young men were nurtured and tutored in lovemaking until, their anxieties diminished and their confidence buoyed, they left her. Mary had cynically trained herself to an expectation that others would have no genuine interest in her feelings, and she had consequently ceased to ask to be heard.

Comment

This case example captures Bowlby's (1977) compulsive caregiving pattern exactly. According to Bowlby (1977, p. 207), "The person showing it may engage in many close relationships but always in the role of giving care, never that of receiving it. . . . The person who develops in this way has found that the only affectional bond available is one in which he must always be the caregiver and the only care he can ever receive is the care he gives himself." In another context, DSM-III-R's self-defeating personality disorder may be seen to encompass this dysfunctional pattern of attachment behaviors.

Mary's interaction with her mother had taught her that deference and subjugation of the self to the other was the price exacted by attachment. In her adult relationships she developed affectional ties along old relational lines: Playing the role of the caregiver was the vehicle through which she sought and maintained relational proximity. Although this accomplished the *set goal* of attachment, the *function* of attachment—to promote safety and security—remained unfulfilled because Mary was not able to satisfy her own attachment needs and to express herself openly and honestly. In relationships, there was painful loneliness for Mary and feelings of yearning and sadness.

Case Example 2

David, aged 33, was a virtual isolate who lived alone with his cat and rarely visited anyone. He sought help for his "shyness and lack of ease around people," although he did not wish to become adept at routine socializing. David was a slim, boyish-looking man with expressive eyes and an awkward, stiff gait.

During childhood the family (parents and an older and younger brother) was the scene of much somberness and some quarreling. His father, a military man described as "aloof and insensitive," emphasized decorum, obedience, respectability, and accepting life whether it was pleasant or not. David noted that his father had "a having your shoes shined philosophy" of life. This atmosphere did not encourage self-expression or self-assertion. There was a deadening quality to home life from which David sought refuge in books. Unfortunately, such interests were denigrated by his father and brothers as "girlish," and equated with women's knitting. David, excluded from the masculine world, felt he lacked the knowledge to succeed in that world. Wistfully, he recalled never having been invited on fishing trips or to play catch with his father and brothers. Further, they delighted in belittling him in front of visitors. He often withdrew to the basement, locked the door, and stayed there until the visitors left.

Rejected by his father and brothers, David sought solace from his mother. She was from a prominent family, one maintained more by a tradition of extreme respectability than by its wealth. Her marriage to David's father was not accepted by her family, who considered him "not one of our kind." Army life necessitated many relocations so that his mother missed the security of the familiar relationships of her family and her hometown friends. Having once felt herself privileged, her reduced status now aroused bitter, dispirited feelings. In David's words, "The most vivid picture I have of my mother is her sitting at the kitchen table staring into space, oblivious to all around her." She appeared to David to be imprisoned by a "circle of sorrow" that he could not penetrate.

Turning to interactions with other children, David, always the loner, hung uncomfortably on the edge of the school playground waiting to be invited to play: "I never tried to push my way in because I felt I had little to offer." Timid, unathletic, and slight of build, David experienced humiliations because physical prowess was all-important: "The kids mimicked my posture and gait." Afraid of children his own age, he kept apart from them. By high school he had "gotten more shy and self-conscious" and — not being ready to take part in social activities — he made no friends.

After completing high school, David attended an out-of-town college that had an excellent liberal arts program. This move was not viewed as an opportunity to cut moorings to home and parents. Instead, he acknowledged that such moves were temporary: "In my mind I knew that I'd always return home." At college, accustomed to reading, studying, thinking, and always giving intellect a significant place in his life, David excelled. Being dispassionate and detached had great appeal to David since feelings were a source of anxiety for him. Through intellectual analysis, old hurts and current sensitivities could not only be put aside but also handled so abstractly that they were neutralized. He began to write poetry in which he himself figured as the central character, thereby turning himself into an object for literary analysis. Later, in therapy, his poems were used as "the royal road" to discover his emotional potentialities.

David was very secretive and reluctant to ask even the most casual questions of other people. His lifelong motto was "Never give yourself away," since the more others knew about him, the more he feared that they would judge him unfairly. In therapy, it became apparent that an intense sensitivity underlay his emotional reserve. He did not tell others much about himself because of his fear that they would use this information to embarrass him. He stayed away from other people for fear of being humiliated, and also because he felt that they would have no genuine interest in him. The implication of this view of others for the therapeutic relationship were explored in terms of such themes as his distrust of the therapist's continuing welcome to him and a feeling of being a burden to the therapist ("You could be doing something more worthwhile with your time").

In social situations, David felt as if his intense anxiety "infected" others and made them nervous just from being around him. Others, perceiving his high anxiety, he felt, would pity him and then patronize him. He spoke of his desire for "someone close who needed me." These longings were revealed by such statements as, "It seems just like it was back in the schoolyard; I'm always on the outside looking in" and "With all the people out there, why doesn't someone find me?" His poems were utilized to reveal his fears and conflicts regarding emotional involvement with others. These poems appeared to offer a second chance to deal with hurtful past events. "I write about aspects of myself that others have ridiculed or aspects of myself that I have hidden from others."

One poem depicted David, in valet fashion, helping his father into his military uniform. Associations revealed themes of subservience and unsuccessful placation of his father. Following this pattern, close relationships appeared to involve the fear of being engulfed in excessive demands and expectations. Another poem indicated strong yearnings for care expressed in the fantasy of being a woman: "If I were a woman, I could be taken care of and not have to make my own way in the world." Earlier, it was noted that moves toward independence were seen by David as temporary. Associations also revealed that returning home was in effect returning to mother; although she was unresponsive, "at least she was always there." Faced with a nonwelcoming, threatening outer world, flight in the form of a return to the secure base of home was stimulated.

Comment

This case example well illustrates Bowlby's (1977) compulsive self-sufficiency pattern. Such pathogenic beliefs about attachment originate from experiences of caregiver responsive failures during childhood. In David's case, he was confronted by a father who dismissed attachment emotions, and who therefore generally failed or refused to recognize David's attachment behaviors. His mother was lost to him through her chronic depression, making her unable to communicate with him in terms of feelings. In fact, David's legitimate feelings of anger and sadness were discouraged by his parents, neither of whom could tolerate such feelings. The consequent view David had of the attachment figure was of one who did not have anything to give. He thus maintained a public self of rigid self-sufficiency "in order to avoid the pain of being rejected," while at the same time "yearning for love and support" (Bowlby, 1977, p. 207).

It is clear that David was personality-disordered. Since childhood he had shown a variety of traits that had led to social difficulties, and significant personal distress. The case history observations indicate a desire for relationships and a fear of rejection that are the putative hallmarks of avoidant personality disorder. Patients with avoidant personality disorder may show these two traits to differing degrees. Even those who are highly avoidant are also highly desirous of close relationships. The conflict between these two opposing qualities created David's distress.

Case Example 3

Joan, in her late 40s, had experienced symptoms of chronic anxiety for more than 10 years. Her primary attachment figure is her husband. She indicates that she feels very close to him and states that "I need him always to be there" such that when he is away she worries about "falling apart" and has to force herself to keep going. Although she stresses that her husband is very understanding and supportive, she reports feeling that nobody will be there "to catch me if I fall." In this vein, she is very fearful of losing him. Although he is in good health, she mentions that she worries about him dying; hardly a day goes by without such thoughts passing through her mind. She also worries about him when he is away. During his absence she feels convinced that something terrible will happen to him. Thus she usually needs to arrange for additional support on these occasions. Joan also becomes very concerned if he is a little late returning from work or from any other trip outside the home, "fearing that something might have happened to him and I'd be totally alone." Joan also speaks of feeling that she relies too much on her husband and expresses the desire to be able to feel "more grown-up." Yet, she perceives her life as so problem-ridden that she *has* to depend on her husband. Thus, she seeks his advice and reassurance about minor, daily decisions.

Most events that lead to an exacerbation of symptoms resonate with underlying expectancies about the potential inaccessibility of her husband. Any loss or death causes a crisis. Even the death of someone vaguely known, such as a distant neighbor or a friend of a friend, precipitates a crisis. Visiting someone in the hospital for a non-life-threatening condition causes Joan intense anxiety that can last for weeks. Under these stressful conditions, Joan responds with intensified care seeking and clings desperately to her husband. A consequence of this heightened care seeking is that alternate coping responses, such as talking about her problems, seeking to understand the meaning of stressful life events, and other cognitive strategies that reduce anxiety and lead to more effective coping, are not attempted and are even actively undermined. Joan simply clings, and thereby elicits sympathetic care rather than helpful assistance.

Case Example 4

Sarah, a woman in her late 30s, like Joan, displayed a pattern of anxious attachment to her husband. She dislikes being alone and feels anxious whenever he is away. She worries about what may happen to her and the children during his absence, and whether they will survive until he returns. Unlike Joan, however, she does not manifest anxiety by worry alone while he is away. She feels intensely resentful about his absence, even when it is due to unavoidable business commitments. Although fearful, she does not show the intense care seeking that characterizes Joan. Instead, she shows a pattern that could best be described as "angry withdrawal." She is unable to express any feelings when her husband returns and does not let him know that she dislikes him being away and that she misses him. Her only response is to withdraw into a sullen, sulky silence. This pattern is manifested most often during times of stress. While Joan responds by showing increased care seeking under these circumstances, Sarah does not actively approach her husband. Although her husband is available, she does not use him for support. He is prepared to listen but she does not inform him of her difficulties or her distress. He is blamed for events that are outside his control and is expected to know, almost magically, without being told, that she is distressed and in need of comfort. This perceived lack of care intensifies her anger and prompts her symptoms to occur, with active coping rarely or unsuccessfully attempted. Whereas Joan is able to use her husband for emotional but not cognitive support, Sarah is unable to use her husband in any way. She feels alone with her problems, and resents this loneliness. This merely intensifies her anger. She abandons attempts to cope with problems in order to punish her husband for their occurrence.

Both Joan and Sarah had typical patterns of dysfunctional parenting that Bowlby (1977) has described as the antecedents of anxious attachment. Joan saw her mother as overprotective and aggressive, giving her little opportunity to grow up and be independent. Her father began to drink when she was about 10 and quarreled frequently with her mother. In response to the increasing marital discord, her mother threatened to abandon the family, out of anger toward her husband. Thereafter, fearing that her mother would make good upon her threat to leave, Joan waited at the bus stop each evening to meet her mother coming home from work. On one occasion, Joan remembered, her mother was late; two or three buses stopped and her mother was not on any of them. Joan was "scared to death" that her mother would never come home again.

Of her family, Sarah said that it was not an affectionate one. Her father was described as "very stern and uncompromising." Sarah consciously hated him during adolescence. There was nothing she could do to win his approval. "He always discouraged me and had such a negative attitude toward me." Although he rarely got overtly angry, her father held grudges and wouldn't speak to her for days. Her mother didn't take her part. In Sarah's eyes, she was a "weakling" whom her father dominated. As well, her mother always seemed to be sick, alleging that she had heart trouble, and warned Sarah constantly that she (the mother) would die if Sarah were "bad."

Comment

The family experiences of Joan and Sarah had led to watchful anxiety as a response to the risk of loss of the caregiver. In their marriages, both similarly feared the loss of security that they had invested in their husbands. Their husband's attention became the index both of them used to judge the relationship's security. But Joan seems to typify a form of anxious attachment in which compulsive care seeking predominates, whereas Sarah—though no less anxious—responds to activation of the attachment system with anger. These last two examples highlight the importance of differentiating the *affective context* associated with attachment patterns.

CONCLUSION

The concept of individuals seeking security and learning in accordance with experiences of the reliability of their attachment figures is the basis for the formulation of many variables of attachment theory. In these clinical examples, we have seen some of the difficulties that may be experienced in forming and sustaining affectional ties. These four individuals showed a wide range of attachment attitudes and behaviors. Can we bring some organization and understanding into the difficulties of relating as diverse as those described in this chapter? What does it mean to be insecurely attached? What sense can be made of the etiological conditions that lead to insecure attachment? The answers to these questions, of course, require that they be framed in relation to secure attachment, for this is the backdrop against which patterns of insecure attachment must be seen. The topics taken up in the subsequent chapters of this book are an attempt to answer these questions and provide a better understanding of the attachment stories presented in this chapter. In Chapter 8, we deal explicitly with the explanatory power of patterns of insecure attachment in relationship to specific personality disorders.

T H R E E
DEVELOPMENTAL PERSPECTIVES

The primary purpose of an attachment relationship, as we
have shown, is the provision of security. This security is
afforded by proximity to a particular individual: in childhood, to a stronger and/or wiser caregiver, and in adulthood, to a peer-partner. The postulate that there are "common
variations" in the way a caregiver responds to the child's attachment behaviors is, of course, central to attachment theory. Early
attachment experiences are the "data" an individual uses to construct a working model of self in relation to others. In this and
the next chapter we shall develop the idea that specific childhood
working models which are carried forward to adulthood have
been given special pressure for continuity through having been
validated by successive attachment experiences. But in order to
do this job, we will first review and compare some of the main
features of the traditional psychoanalytic and attachment models
of development.

TRADITIONAL PSYCHOANALYTIC THEORY

Virtually all psychoanalytic theorists stress that important experiences from the past are transferred to the present. This view
of the past as transferred to the psychological present is related
as well to the psychoanalytical emphasis upon the fixity of inner
structures. To find the past in the present, then, not only requires
detecting traces of remote events beneath current relational realities, but also noting "unfinished business" — unfulfilled needs that

were initiated in childhood, but which still organize present processes.

Considerations of this kind about development are the most characteristic feature of the traditional psychoanalytic approach to psychopathology and, as we shall see, of the object relations approach as well. For purposes of exposition, we confine our overview to the developmental model that has its roots most directly in the work of Freud. We want to emphasize the following six components. These components by no means completely capture the psychoanalytic model, or even necessarily represent the foundational elements of the model. They are emphasized in this context because of their relevance as contrasts to Bowlby's formulations.

1. Behaviors are fueled by "nervous or physical energy." In the last half of the nineteenth century, the greater share of scientific enquiry was directed toward the study of physical energy: its forms, laws, and measurement. Freud framed his theories within an energy model, speaking of the discharge, inertia, and constancy of psychical energy.

2. The personality is organized to control dangerous primitive instinctual drives, notably aggression and sexuality. In the same way in which elaborated social institutions within advanced cultures constrain and "civilize" mankind in general, so the elaborated structures of the ego and superego within the individual constrain and "civilize" the primitive id.

3. Normal development follows a single predictable pathway, through landmark achievements. Pathological development occurs when an individual fails to achieve a significant landmark; all subsequent landmarks are affected by this failure.

4. Failure to achieve a landmark is generally the consequence of specific events or interactions. Traditionally, the psychoanalytic approach involves the reconstruction of past events to uncover the causes that *overdetermine* current behaviors.

5. Failure to achieve a landmark affects all further development; that is, it leaves an encapsulated-like residue of infantile fixations. These residues are *frozen* within the individual's character structure and consequently continue to operate irrespective of other causes for continuance.

6. The primary danger or threat is punishment; that is, some form of retribution or untoward consequence for failing to control and civilize primitive drives.

In summary, traditional psychoanalytic theory depicts a single route to normality. Each stage on this journey builds on previous stages. If at some stage normal development is interfered with by some adverse experience or experiences, then all subsequent stages are affected and normal development is precluded. In Figure 3.1 we have represented this model of development as an inverted pyramid, with each stage of development being more highly differentiated than the previous stage, but resting of necessity on all previous stages. According to this model, any missing or malformed component of a foundational stage will promote instability in all further developmental stages. If a foundational stage is too severely malformed, then the later stages may collapse downward.

OBJECT RELATIONS THEORY

The view of development, from the perspective of object relations theorists, often adds up to about the same thing. Both psychoanalysts and members of the object relations school agree that development proceeds in a sequential fashion in which processes unfold naturally. Growth toward such objectives as mature dependence (Fairbairn, 1952), libidinal object constancy (Mahler et al., 1975), and coherent selfhood (Kohut, 1971) is regarded as an orderly linear psychic development. And what prevents development? The treatments of the child by its caregivers play a crucial role in the object relations theory of psychological disturbance. Parental provisions that do not adequately meet the child's needs result in arrested development: the child does not move forward, but instead becomes frozen. Continuity with the past is accented. Needs unmet in childhood, buried because this was the only means for adapting to environmental failure, persist and await expression. Although the language and imagery of the traditional psychoanalytic and object relations models are

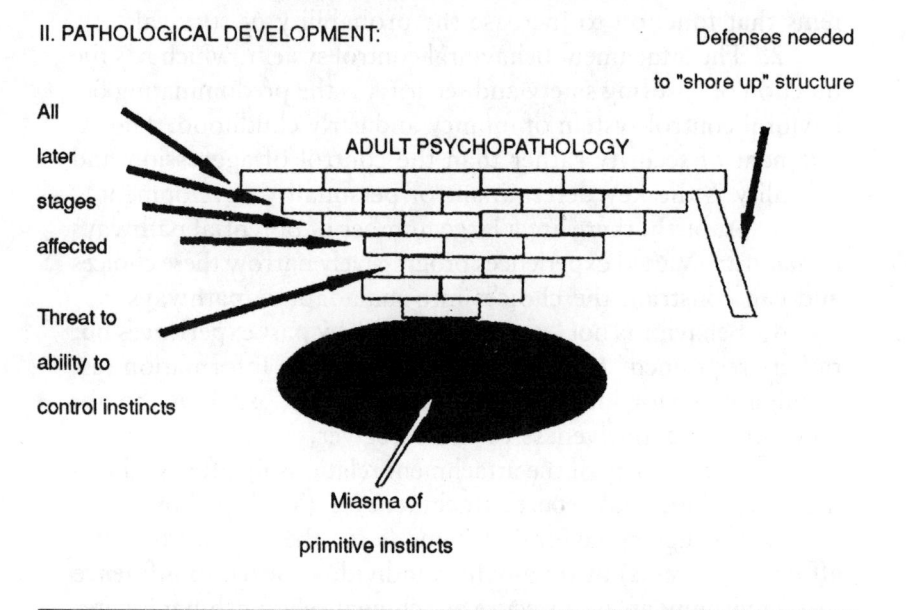

I. NORMAL DEVELOPMENT:

ADULT MATURITY

Stages of
personality
development

Adaptive
mechanisms for
controlling
primitive
instincts

Miasma of

primitive instincts

II. PATHOLOGICAL DEVELOPMENT:

Defenses needed
to "shore up" structure

All
later
stages
affected

ADULT PSYCHOPATHOLOGY

Threat to
ability to
control instincts

Miasma of

primitive instincts

FIGURE 3.1. Orthodox Psychoanalytic Theory of Development.

clearly different, both models depict adult relationships as fixed residues from early childhood experiences.

In the above models of development, early adaptations remain like wounds in the trunk of a tree; all future growth must go around them. And as wounds, they are susceptible to reopening, thus also affecting future growth.

ATTACHMENT THEORY

The six points presented here illustrate the fundamentals of Bowlby's theory of development and correspond to the six points summarizing the Freudian approach presented earlier in this chapter.

1. Behaviors are determined by the set goals of control systems that function to increase the probability of survival.

2. The attachment behavioral control system, which has the function of ensuring safety and security, is the predominating behavioral control system of infancy and early childhood. The attainment of security rather than the control of aggression and sexuality is the key determinant of personality development.

3. At birth, there are a large number of potential pathways to maturity. Varied experiences progressively narrow these choices and can constrain the choices into maladaptive pathways.

4. Behavior is not "overdetermined" by past experiences but rather "restrained" from alternative pathways. Information restraining behavior includes "zero information," such as the absence or unresponsiveness of the caregiver.

5. The security of the attachment relationship affects all further development. A secure attachment relationship allows activation of other behavioral systems (e.g., the exploratory and affiliative systems) through which individuals learn to influence their environment. An insecure attachment relationship mitigates against full expression of other behavioral systems.

6. The primary danger or threat is loss of the attachment figure (cf. distance from the attachment figure for infants).

Unlike traditional psychoanalytic and object relations theories of development, attachment theory gets along without any stages of development at all, at least when it is directed to the issue of the continuity or discontinuity of different patterns of attachment. To be sure, the capacity to form an attachment bond to a caregiver follows a phase-specific course and exhibits characteristics peculiar to each phase. Insofar, then, as we conceive of these attachment variants as the manifestation of a particular phase, we may speak of the growth of attachment. Once the pre-attachment phases are past (generally by age 12 to 18 months), and an attachment relationship has been achieved, discrete attachment patterns evolve from the outcomes of attachment experiences in which the child's age plays no part. This is another way of saying that different attachment patterns have their source in a dyadic relationship without being tied to any endogenous phase of development, as is the case in the traditional psychoanalytic account of psychosexual development, to take the most obvious and well-known example.

ATTACHMENT DEVELOPMENT OVER THE LIFE SPAN

According to traditional psychoanalytic theory, the infant becomes attached to the mother as a result of her ability to satisfy the infant's physiological needs. These needs, directed first toward the caregiver and later toward others, are increasingly expressed in more or less acceptable ways. But this social control is not won without a struggle. Even after the child has become attached to the mother, the drives tend to persist in their original form. Inner conflict results as the child adopts more complex arrangements to obtain gratification of basic needs while at the same time avoiding anxiety or warding off punishment. Schafer (1983, p. 213) proposed using the metaphor of the infant as beast to capture Freud's account of this unfolding of development: "One of the primary narrative structures begins with the infant and young child as a beast, otherwise known as the id, and ends with the beast domesticated, tamed by frustration in the course of development in a civilization hostile to its nature."

Bowlby's attachment infant has a very different nature. This infant is not innately driven by socially unacceptable urges, but

41

rather inherently predisposed to behaviors that promote proximity to others. Unlike Freud's infant who is driven by the seeking of oral pleasure, the attachment infant is born with a behavioral control system activated by threats to safety and security and expressed in behaviors such as clinging, crying, following, and smiling, all of which play a critical part in the making of a strong affectional tie with the caregiver. Basic instinctual responses on one side and loving availability on the other create the reciprocal patterning of interaction for the formation of the child's first affectional bond. Bowlby (1958, p. 364) summarizes this key idea:

> It is my thesis that, as in the young of other species, there matures in the early months of life of the human infant a complex and nicely balanced equipment of instinctual responses, the function of which is to ensure that he obtains parental care sufficient for his survival. To this end the equipment includes responses which promote his close proximity to a parent and responses which evoke parental activity.

All these components, then, contribute to a relationship that is critical to the child's early sense of felt security.

Winnicott, who was a colleague of Bowlby's, reached much the same conclusions about the primacy and long-lasting effects of the child–mother relationship without recourse to the ethological and evolutionary requirements that were the foundation of Bowlby's theory. In his paper "The Capacity to Be Alone," Winnicott (1965, p. 31) described the nature of the parental holding environment that creates what he called ego-relatedness:

> Although many types of experience go to the establishment of the capacity to be alone, there is one that is basic, and without a sufficiency of it the capacity to be alone does not come about; this experience is that of being alone, as an infant and a young child, in the presence of mother. Thus the basis of the capacity to be alone is a paradox; it is the experience of being alone while someone else is present.

According to this quote, we could not say that Winnicott and Bowlby differed with respect to the kinds of experiences that promote a secure relational foundation. Although inclined to focus on the consequences of parental impingement to the child's sense of selfhood, Winnicott's study of the self is embedded in the context of the caregiver's empathetic responsiveness.[1]

Bowlby's story line has served attachment researchers as an indispensable code for comparative accounts of attachment development in terms of different beginnings, course, and outcome. Mary Ainsworth used this general code as the basis for a rating system to distinguish qualitatively different attachment relationships between infants and mothers. These studies have become landmarks in the literature on infant attachment. For this reason, and because her work impacts on the issue of how much of the past is to be found in the present, we will examine this research in some detail.

Ainsworth and her colleagues have characterized attachment bonds in infants through systematic observation of specific behaviors for maintaining proximity (e.g., clinging), reestablishing proximity (e.g., reaching, following), protesting separation (e.g., crying), and demonstrating pleasure in reunion (e.g., smiling, physical contact). To identify and classify these attachment behaviors, a laboratory procedure known as the Strange Situation Protocol was developed (Ainsworth & Wittig, 1969). Because of the predominance of the attachment system in infancy, the behaviors are evoked by a very mild stressor (brief separation from the caregiver in a safe environment). Within a controlled setting a 1-year-old infant is briefly separated from his or her primary caregiver, visited by a stranger, and then reunited with the caregiver in a precisely prescribed sequence of eight stages. The infant's behaviors on separation from and reunion with the caregiver and in the presence of the stranger are used to define four general patterns of attachment relationships: secure, avoidant, ambivalent, and disorganized. Because Ainsworth's patterns are prominent in the attachment literature, we will only describe them here very briefly.

Secure infants, labeled Group B, showed the most adaptive behaviors in the situation. They greeted the mother upon reunion with smiles, vocalization, waving, and/or by seeking physical contact. The avoidant infants, labeled Group A, showed avoidance of proximity during reunion with the parent, turning away or simply ignoring the mother. Another group of infants, ambivalent infants, labelled Group C, sought contact with the mother upon reunion, but they were also conspicuously resistant and angry in their reaction to her. Infants classified as disorganized, Group D, failed to exhibit a consistent strategy on activation of the attachment system but instead showed a pronounced mixture of both patterns of insecure attachment and may have exhibited entirely extraneous behavioral responses. This disorganized pattern was recognized as a discrete and consistent behavioral pattern at a later date than the other three patterns (Main & Solomon, 1987).

Internalization

While Schafer used the metaphor of the beast to capture Freud's story line of the infant, Bowlby's portrayal of the infant gives rise to an alternate story line. As developed by Bowlby, the attachment infant is impelled instinctively to form a bond with a caregiver, usually the mother. When security is threatened, the child seeks closer proximity to the caregiver. If all goes well and the child experiences appropriate responsiveness from the caregiver (i.e., the caregiver aids and abets the child's proximity-seeking), then closer physical proximity is achieved, the sense of threat diminishes, and security is reestablished. Over time, successive experiences of this sort build internalized attitudes and beliefs about the self and others; that is, *working models* of others as available and of the self as worthy of care and effective in eliciting care.

But if all does not go well and the attachment figure ignores, rebuffs, or punishes the child's proximity-seeking, then attachment behaviors do *not* lead to closer physical proximity. The original threat is not diminished, and a new threat accrues: the threat of loss of the necessary relationship. Because the attachment system uses environmental feedback to assess goal attainment, the child with an inadequately responsive attachment figure is caught in a double bind. Threats to security dictate proximity-seeking behaviors; the attachment figure's (unsatisfactory) response to proximity-seeking further threatens security and therefore dictates *both* increased proximity-seeking (because security is further threatened) and a cessation of proximity-seeking (because feedback information confirms that proximity-seeking is counterproductive to the goal of proximity)! This threat is handled by a defensive organization of the attachment system, giving rise to patterns of insecure attachment. In Bowlby's story each of us comes to be located at some point along a spectrum ranging from secure to insecure attachment.

The actual experiences within the caregiver–child relationship (that is, the degree of success in having needs met) thus become the basis for an internalized representation of attachment. Continued lack of success in achieving felt security forms the basis for a representation of attachment as unproductive or insecure.

Continuity

According to attachment theory, then, caregiver responsiveness failures are transferred to the child's inner representational world. As suggested by Main et al. (1985), what is internalized is the child-in-relation-to-the-attachment-figure, rather than the attachment figure per se, creating a cognitive / affective schema of this first attachment relationship. Specific attitudes, expectations, and feelings toward attachment that persist into later age periods, including adulthood, are not, however, the direct result of early working models that are common to Ainsworth's infant attachment patterns. Instead, working models persist when they encounter attachment strains of a quality and intensity consistent with the child's earliest attachment experiences. In other words, when subsequent attachment events reinforce the child's working model, making it painfully real and accurate in the instance of noxious caregiver responses, the organizing potential is particularly powerful. It is this confirmation of early working models in the form of later attachment experiences that contribute to their persistence.

Thus, an understanding of tendencies in the representational world that persist through time and enter into the determination of later attachment issues requires more rather than less attention to individuals' ongoing relationship matrix. This emphasis on successive attachment experiences interacting with prior experiences, through the representational world, to determine the individual's current state of mind with regards to attachment is consistent with post-Freudian writers such as Kris's (1956) and Khan's (1963) concepts of "strain" and "cumulative" trauma. It is generally agreed that the lack of empathetic care or, to use Stern's (1985) term, the lack of the caregiver's *affect attunement* to the child, can disrupt as surely as an acute environmental trauma such as abuse or the death of a parent. Strain trauma broadens the idea of loss to include long-repeated and partial losses such as the chronic inability of the caregiver to relate sensitively to the child. Parentification of the child or life with a depressed parent, examples offered by Bowlby (1977) of deficits and failures of the caregiver's accessibility, can be regarded as strain traumas. In fact, the frightening effect of abuse may result as much from the loss of the parent as a source of comfort, thereby engendering in the child a feeling of being alone and, hence, an experience of helplessness, than from the acute impact of the abuse itself (Main & Hesse, 1990).

As we have seen, psychoanalytic thinking about development has, by and large, adhered to the view that fixity of relational functioning derives from early childhood experiences. While attachment writers have also been concerned with early experiences as a source of continuity, they have equally accented the role of ongoing family experiences for the persistence of a developmental pathway. As an example of stability of attachment patterns in early childhood, we may consider the work of Main and Cassidy (1988).

These investigators focused on a group of parents and children who had been assessed in the Strange Situation Protocol at 12 months and then reassessed when the children were 6 years of age. Confining our attention to the avoidantly attached children (Ainsworth's Group A infants), strong evidence for the stability of avoidance emerged from these studies. For example, 75% of the children classified as avoidant of mother as infants were also avoidant of her at age 6. If we further take into account the finding that a reliable correlation has been demonstrated between avoidant infants and dismissing mothers (those individuals for whom the importance of attachment emotions and relations is minimal), then we may argue that caregiver responsiveness failures are not under most circumstances limited to any specific time period in the child's life. As Bowlby (1973, p. 368) suggests:

> Environmental pressures are due largely to the fact that the family environment in which a child lives and grows tends to remain relatively unchanged. . . . This means that whatever family pressures led the development of a child to take the pathway he is now on are likely to persist and so to maintain development on that same pathway.

Thus, it seems reasonable to assume that the dismissing mother who was uncomfortable with her infant "sinking into" (Ainsworth et al., 1978) her might also be unavailable to negotiate and develop mutually agreeable plans with a 6-year-old and fail to be an "attachment figure in reserve" (Weiss, 1991) for the adolescent. In an essential way, then, relational themes and problems may be the same (or very similar) across the attachment history of the child, varying only in how they are expressed at different ages. Although an avoidant pattern of attachment, for example, may begin in infancy, the quality of parent–child interactions from which it arose are not intrinsic to these early years, but rather are just as likely to typify interactions in later childhood and adolescence as well. This attachment perspective is an important antidote to those versions of psychopathology in which everything of consequence is tied to fixations of the earliest developmental needs. Patterns of insecure attachment are, therefore, perhaps best viewed as strategies for coping with a difficult interpersonal world learned over the course of infancy to adolescence.

If an individual tells an attachment story of an unfortunate and troublesome pattern of relating that has endured for years, we also need to consider another source of continuity: durable personality structures that do not easily yield to change. As Bowlby (1973, p. 369) points out:

> Structural features of personality once developed, have their own means of self-regulation that tend also to maintain the current direction of development. For example, present cognitive or behavioral structures determine what is perceived and what ignored, how a situation is construed, and what

plan of action is likely to be constructed to deal with it. Current structures, moreover, determine what sorts of person and situation are sought after and what sorts are shunned. In this way an individual comes to influence the selection of his own environment; and so the wheel comes full circle.

Starting with the indisputable fact that the child is enmeshed in a relational network and that nothing about his or her personality development can be fully understood apart from this interactional context, Bowlby borrowed the biologist Waddington's theory of epigenetic developmental pathways. This way of looking at development is neatly stated in Waddington's own words (1957, p. 189):

> Organism and environment are not two separate things, each having its own character in its own right, which come together with little essential interrelation as a sieve and a shovelful of pebbles thrown on to it. The fundamental characteristics of the organism are time-extended properties, which can be envisaged as a set of alternative pathways of development.

In this model, there is no single route to normality. Attachment experiences constrain the choice among possible alternatives rather than blocking further development. Additionally, the great benefit of the notion of alternative pathways is that continuity of development is accounted for by "time-extended properties" of the organism, while at the same time it allows for the possibility of new beginnings that can alter the course of a pathway. Following Bowlby's lead, we have used Waddington's imagery to model this developmental paradigm in Figure 3.2. The great tree of development lies on its side; we each begin with the common trunk of biological species and birth. But individual differences in genetics and environment constrain us to follow different limbs of the tree. As our experiences elaborate, so our path continues to divide from other possible paths, so that in the end, each person resides on an individual twig which can, nonetheless, be traced back through increasingly common branches to the main trunk.

In this view, early attachment experiences do not leave

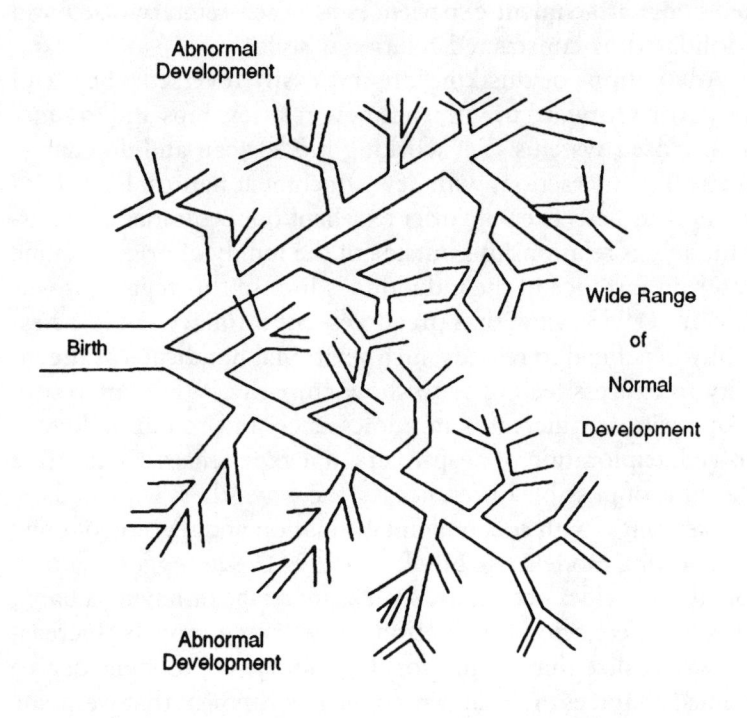

Abnormal
Development

Birth

Wide Range

of

Normal

Development

Abnormal
Development

FIGURE 3.2. Bowlby's Theory of Development. In this model, development is not blocked by particular experiences of deficits, but rather is constrained into increasingly particular pathways. There is no "royal road" to normality; rather, there are numerous pathways, or branches, that cluster within the normal range.

psychoanalytic-like residues that are transferred to new relationships, but instead provide a kind of relational chart for managing current relationships. Childhood attachment experiences are internalized, thereafter become the basis for the earliest representations of attachment, and thereby determine relational patterns. Put simply, what was external (child–caregiver interactions) is internalized and then projected afterward onto subsequent experiences. Once projected onto new relationships, further disappointment and frustration of attachment desires are likely to accrue. These attachment experiences are then reinternalized and consolidated as constricted relational styles.

Adaptations of this kind are not easily reversed; they tend to be carried forward to influence new relationships and to function as closed systems. Yet working models can and do change as a result of interactions with new attachment figures. Late childhood and adolescence may offer excellent opportunities for revising models as relationships outside of the family of origin assume greater importance in the individual's life. In this regard, it was Sullivan's (1953) view that preadolescent intimacy could be especially beneficial to remedy such relational handicaps as the inability to express feeling or to show empathy. When interest in the opposite sex increases in adolescence and romantic love is involved, exploration of deeply personal experiences can increase awareness of possible differences in the way others view and experience things, with concomitant evaluation and revision of one's own working models. As Bowlby (1969/1982) suggests, adulthood also provides occasions, such as marriage or having a baby, that require conscious evaluations of working models. Increasingly, we realize that if our working models are to some degree sustained by forces in the interpersonal environment that we create for ourselves, they may also be altered by some major changes in this environment.

Unfortunately, adaptations made under conditions of attachment strain are not easily changed, particularly if, as is so often the case during childhood and adolescence, the strains are continuing. The long-term effect of early attachment experiences upon later peer relationships is dramatically evidenced in Tizard and Hodge's (1978) study of institution-reared children. These children had been institutionally reared for the first 4 years of their lives and subsequently either adopted or restored to their biological family. Although the adopted and restored children differed with regard to their family circumstances (the adoptive children appeared to have warm and supportive homes while those of the restored children were troublesome and discordant), both groups as adolescents showed poorer social relations than did their matched controls. Finally, various studies of the intergenerational transmission of attachment patterns indicate that the majority of mothers do not break the cycle of passing on the effects of unhappy attachment experiences to their own children (e.g., Crowell & Feldman, 1988; Grossmann, Fremmer-Bombik, Rudolph, & Grossmann, 1988; Main & Goldwyn, 1984; Ricks, 1985).

Considerations of this kind can easily lead one to agree with Oscar Wilde that we are our past and that through our representational world we are carried along by this past. Woody Allen, who is a keen observer of psychoanalysis, expressed a similar theme in the movie *Crimes and Misdemeanors:*

> You will notice that what we are aiming at when we fall in love is a very strange paradox. The paradox consists of the fact that when we fall in love, we are seeking to refind all or some of the people to whom we were attached as children. On the other hand, we ask our beloved to correct all of the wrongs that these early parents or siblings inflicted upon us. So that love contains in it the contradiction; the attempts to *return* to the past and the attempts to *undo* the past.

Working Model

In simplified terms, the actual experiences of a caregiver's *availability* accumulate to form, on the one hand, *expectations* about the reliability of attachment, and, on the other hand, *self-concepts* about one's ability to evoke attachment responses. In addition to these cognitive components, these set representations encompass a pattern of affects throughout the individual's life. Not infrequently, a single affect may be central to the individual's model. The major feelings that are intertwined and become especially a part of insecure representations of attachment are anger, yearning, anxiety, guilt, and sadness. From the discussion of the dynamics of insecure attachment that we take up in a later chapter, it will be apparent that such feelings are associated ultimately with the anticipated and expected loss of the current attachment figure.

The important point just now is to appreciate the role these inner representations play in maintaining an individual's relational pathway. Expectations about present attachment relationships are associated with a comparison of things in the present with the individual's representational world. Perceptions of the current attachment figure are filtered through a model of past attachment experiences. In this sense, an individual's model of attachment and of self is guided by its own rules. These rules have, on the one hand, the obvious advantage of lending a certain coherence to the conception of attachment. Yet, on the other hand, there is the possibility that the rules may tend to harden into rigid attitudes toward self and attachment, making the individual ignore those aspects of attachment reality that do not fit the model. When the individual's inner representations crystallize into these rigid rules for the passage of attachment information, it may be said to be marked by a decrease in its "permeability." As Bowlby (1977, p. 209) notes, the individual tends "to assimilate any new person with whom he may form a bond to an existing model . . . and often to continue to do so despite repeated evidence that the model is inappropriate." In the next chapter, we characterize the content and process of these inner representations as organized into a working model of attachment relationships.

FOUR

REPRESENTATIONAL OR WORKING MODELS

MENTAL REPRESENTATIONS

Object relations and social cognition[1] writers alike agree that mental representations of the self and other enter into the determination of all interpersonal behavior. The adjustment and psychological health of the individual is often discussed in terms of abstracted features of this representational world, features such as differentiation, integration, richness, and rigidity. Generally, these formal aspects of representational model are not generally matters of theoretical dispute; there is widespread agreement, for example, that the progressive development of representations is primarily a matter of an increase in differentiation. Disagreement exists concerning when and how such differentiation occurs.

Contemporary writing about mental representations appears to have heeded Rapaport's (1959) call for an integration of psychoanalysis with Werner's (1948) treatment of development from a gestalt point of view. Gestalt concepts have become a part of the general culture of psychology and have been used to provide a kind of formal structure of representations. Psychoanalytic theorists have, in effect, filled in these representations with various contents. In Kernberg's (1980) scheme, for example, we see movement from undifferentiated selfobject representations to mature, ambivalent representations. Similarly, Kohut (1971) described the development of a coherent self from a bipolar self, which in turn developed from an early fragmented self. Operational reformulations of psychoanalytic concepts—by Horowitz (1987, 1988), Blatt and Lerner (1983), and Westen (1990), for example—involve stating representations of self and others in terms that allow confirmation or refutation by empirical testing. Many of these reformulations of psychoanalytic ideas about representations can be found in the earlier work of Sandler and Rosenblatt (1962).

BOWLBY'S USE OF REPRESENTATION

Following Craik's (1943) idea of a mental model as a determining tendency of human functioning, Bowlby (1969/1982) introduced the concept of an "internal working model." The choice of this concept appears to have derived from his interest in the practical problem of understanding persistent relational differences among people. As we noted in Chapter 1, later writers in the field of attachment have used the terms "representational model" and "working model" interchangeably. Bowlby expressed a preference for the term "working model" because, to him, it emphasized the continuing active role of these internalized models in controlling the expression of certain behaviors. Both terms encompass the same idea. The working model has been conceived as a skeleton outline or an organized abstraction through which attachment-relevant information is "filtered." It is a self-creation of the individual based on historical experiences with actual attachment figures.

Peterfreund (1983, p. 81) remarked, "At the present time working models are not exact rigorously defined concepts." Under the broadest definition, working model refers to the internal organization of memory, knowledge, experiences, and affects into a coherent whole that can direct and influence evaluations and actions. Similar concepts are important components of psychoanalytic thinking (e.g., Klein, 1958; Slap & Saykin, 1983), cognitive psychology (e.g., Heil, 1983; Neisser, 1976), and the field of artificial intelligence (e.g., Bobrow & Collins, 1975; Hofstadter, 1979).

REPRESENTATIONAL DIFFERENTIATION

As noted above, the degree of *representational differentiation* is the fundamental factor characterizing organized perceptions of self, others, and relationships. Werner (1948) noted that the concept of differentiation can be dealt with on a number of different levels. First, it means a general change in the mode of experience; for example, from brief stores of past experiences that contribute expectations and learned responses in childhood to the pervasiveness of the representational world in adulthood. This difference is reflected in the way representations function to modify the proximity requirement in attachment. In infancy and early childhood termination of activation of the attachment system occurs with physical proximity to the primary caregiver. Repeated experiences with the principal caregiver in childhood are converted into cognitive *schemata,* which permit generalization from past experiences to the present and allow "proximity" to be maintained through cognitive constructs as well as through physical reality. These cognitive schemata are associated with the affects accompanying proximity and, with the addition of such affective content, become working models of the attachment relationship. In the adult, the maintenance of proximity to the attachment figure becomes largely an internalized representational process.

Second, many writers have noted that with development, representations are transformed from vague, diffuse experiences to well-defined ones. Although attachment theory's depiction of working models does not pay much attention to the structural dimension of representations, the growth of representational differentiation is implicit in both Bowlby's and Ainsworth's accounts of the development of the attachment bond.[2] During the first 2 months of life the infant's attachment behaviors are not directed predominantly toward any specific figure. In the "attachment-in-the-making" phase (occurring between 2 and 3 months), discrimination of one or more attachment figures is evident. By 6 months, "clear-cut attachment" is shown by the infant, who maintains proximity to a primary attachment figure through locomotion and signaling. Although this phase is prelinguistic, the child appears to have developed a set of expectations about the responsiveness of the attachment figure; their interactions have an "afterlife" in the form of a beginning working model of the relationship with the parent.

This emerging ability of the child to form enduring models of caregiver–child interactions becomes especially manifest in the phase Bowlby (1969/1982) calls a "goal-corrected partnership." Supported by language and perspective-taking abilities, the older child is able to appreciate the attachment figure as someone with her own plans and goals. Separations, because they can now be planned and mutually understood, are less likely to be felt by the child as threats to the relationship. Additionally, representations have the capacity to supplement actual interactions with the caregiver. In Schafer's (1983) words, representations are "felt presences" within the child that allow children to maintain secure models of their attachment figures even during their physical absence. Thus, from the undifferentiated "attachment-in-the-making" phase emerges a more highly differentiated internal representational capacity that enables the child to affectively cope with separations from the attachment figure.

Third, increased differentiation and self-awareness go together. When Mary Main (1991) speaks of varying ability among people to integrate and discuss attachment information in the context of the Adult Attachment Interview (AAI) (George, Kaplan, & Main, 1985), she may have in mind the idea that complexity of representational content increases the possibility for self-reflection. For instance, the phenomenon of splitting "good" and "bad" experiences with a parent into separate representations (the basis of what Bowlby [1969/1982] terms "multiple models" of attachment figures) decreases consciousness of conflicted feelings about the same individual. This state can be characterized as the impermeability of boundaries separating representations, permitting minimal integration, and therefore lessening the freedom for reflection and understanding.

Fourth, increasing differentiation implies a timetable for its development. Object relations theorists, by and large, have clung to the idea that growth in representational differentiation is rooted in a sequential range of developmental stages with different junctures accomplished in a given time. The developmental target of multidimensional, differentiated representations was thought by object relations theorists to have been attained at age 5 (the oedipal age). Here, as much as in any area of psychoanalysis, conceptual certitude existed in the absence of empirical indexes of the hypothesized timetable for the development of differentiated representations. That such representations are not fully formed until the individual reaches early adolescence is attested to by developmental research carried out during the past 10 years (e.g., Harter 1983, 1986). As summarized by Westen (1990), this work refuted the object relations notion that the oedipal-age period is the seat of complex and subtle representations of self and others.

Fifth, in accordance with Tomkins (1961), most writers stress the importance of affects in accounting for changes in the degree of differentiation of representations. There is more or less general agreement that representations change (become less differentiated and more primitive) as a result of strong affective arousal. For example, in the AAI, the insecure individual's use of "splitting" or dissociation of "good" and "bad" representations of the parents is an indication of difficulties with affect regulation. Apparently, the arousal of strong feelings during the interview undermines the individual's ability to abstract, integrate, or unite concepts of the parents into a coherent representation. In general, affects contribute content to the working model; they are part of the feedback information that modifies its expression and thereby play a significant role in determining the pattern of attachment. As we describe below, the content of the representational world is never affect-free. Moreover, the affectively charged beliefs about attachment embedded in this world are carried forward as potentials to be triggered in current relationships.

COGNITIVE SCHEMA

The working model construct has been closely related to the cognitive concept of *schema* (Rumelhart, 1980). Immanuel Kant first proposed the idea of schemata as part of the process through which data from our senses is converted to information, or knowledge, for our intellect (Aquila, 1983; Kant, 1781; Schiffer

& Steele, 1988). Kant proposed that we use 12 natural or "inborn" categories to understand what the senses perceive; these categories include cause and effect, negation, unity, and totality. In Kant's system, schemata were the rules governing the application of these categories. Schemata, in modern epidemiological parlance, are the inclusion and exclusion criteria for membership in a category. So, for instance, one important schema with which we make sense of our world may be stated simply as, "All causes have effects." In the Kantian system, it would not make sense—nor would it occur naturally—to place a perception in the category of *cause* if it was not matched to a perception that fit the category of *effect*.

The concept of schemata becomes more closely related to the concept of working model in its twentieth century development by Henry Head (1926) and Frederic Bartlett (1932). Bartlett, in particular, elaborated Kantian schemata to model how human memory operates. Memory, according to Bartlett, does not access a simple museum of past experiences, where each experience is preserved in its "true" original form. Rather, memory creates a kind of story, using some historically accurate details, some partially accurate and partially reconstructed details, and some wholly fabricated details. No longer abbreviated "criteria" as in the Kantian system, in Bartlett's model schemata evolved into the "plausible scenarios" that we use to construct these stories, supplying both the general outline to follow and, as necessary, missing details and information to complete the story. Current psychoanalytic writers seem to take this same view of the matter, arguing that reconstruction of the analysand's past is not a question of "finding out what really happened" (historical truth) but a matter of eliciting "narrative fit" (Schafer, 1983; Spence, 1982).

The great advantage that schemata offer is the ability to operate with incomplete, fragmentary, and even contradictory information (Ayer, 1946; Kempson, 1988). But this advantage can turn into a disadvantage when what is required of us is not recognition of old patterns but acceptance of a perception that does not fit old patterns. The West Indies are so named because Christopher Columbus's schema, dominated by the belief that the world was round and *small,* did not allow for another continent between Europe and Asia. When he reached land after sailing from Spain, his most plausible scenario (i.e., schema) was that this land was India; hence the name of the islands in the Caribbean and the appellation of "Indians" for the original inhabitants of the entire land. History is replete with examples of the disastrous consequences of retaining outmoded schemata.

In the words of Campbell (1989, pp. 95–96):

> [Schemata] put together whole tracts of knowledge out of a scattering of parts, amplify and extend impoverished data, and make sense of what seems to be nonsense. Schemata guide us through the thickets of complexity that confront us at every waking moment. . . . [But] as aids to action, they are apt to anchor us in the mundane, the plausible, the familiar and they are ruthless in the way they murder possibilities, cutting a path along which we can move in confidence without being diverted by alternative routes.

One major modification is needed in the concept of schemata in order to arrive at working models. Schemata belong to the cognitive domain, converting perceptions to knowledge and enabling decisions and actions based on knowledge. Working models include knowledge but are most closely concerned with converting discrete behavioral interactions into relationships and evoking emotional responses based on relationships. Schemata organize information; working models organize relationships. To use a physical metaphor: Imagine an abstract painting inspired by the biblical story of the Prodigal Son. An analogue to a *schema* would be the title of *A Farmer's Son Returns Home;* an analogue to a *working model* would be the title *An Anxious Son Hopes for Forgiveness from a Loving Father.* Both titles predispose the viewer to a specific interpretation of the painting; but the second title focuses on the emotional relationship rather than the organizing facts. Working models can be considered a special class of schema, namely, a class of schema that encodes affective as well as cognitive information.

THE "TRADITIONAL" UNDERSTANDING
OF THE ATTACHMENT SYSTEM'S WORKING MODEL

The *representational* or *working model* is a mechanism of development and continuity across the life span (Bowlby, 1988b; Sroufe, 1986). From earliest infancy a young child has repeated experiences that contain at least one similar element: A need is felt and expressed. The consequences of these repeated experiences include the formation and perseverance of a working model.

It is through the working model that the emotions evoked by past attachment experiences are translated into patterns of behavior that largely influence current attachment experiences. Current experiences can, in turn, be incorporated into and modify the existing model. The attachment system of the adult thus contains, through the single mechanism of the working model, the capability for both rigidity and flexibility.

Using this conception of the working model, we can construct a fairly straightforward etiology for adult attachment patterns. Based on his or her early attachment experiences, each individual creates a model of attachment. This model determines the individual's expectations regarding the security of the relationship, and the responsive availability of the attachment figure, based on memories of the attachment figure. The model also contains predispositions to certain affective and behavioral responses to an attachment figure, based on memories of the self in the primal attachment relationship. In other words, from our early attachment experiences we learn what to expect from ourselves and others, we learn the likely affective sequelae of attachment interactions, and we learn behavioral repertoires that seem necessary to maintain or reestablish security. All of these features are encapsulated in a working model, as Bowlby conceives it, to which individuals turn to direct and understand current attachment relationships.

When experience has led an individual to develop a working model of attachment relationship as secure, then that model not only encompasses a responsive attachment figure, a competent self, and appropriate behaviors and affects, but is also subject to revision and adjustment in response to current, new attachment experiences. In Piagetian terms, such working models can accommodate to new information (Piaget, 1954).

When, on the other hand, experience leads an individual to develop a working model of attachment relationships as insecure, then the opposite effects accrue. In these instances, the model encompasses an inadequately responsive attachment figure, an incompetent self (at least in the sphere of attachment), and maladaptive behaviors and affects. Additionally, such insecurity is associated with working models that are rigid and unadaptable. In Piagetian terms, such working models assimilate all new information under old guidelines or rules, regardless of how inaccurately. It is in this sense that Main et al. (1985) speak of the "rules" guiding the attachment system and adult attachment behaviors. This emphasis on "rules" and "structured processes" suggests a view of the working model as an *algorithm:* a set of rules, processes, or steps for solving "attachment problems."

The working model is the primary feature of the adult attachment system (Bowlby, 1988b; Hinde, 1982; Main et al., 1985; Weiss, 1982; Bretherton, 1985). The adult's working model of attachment is based on varied, cumulative, and disjointed attachment experiences. It operates as a component of a larger system of models for different types of relationships, which themselves are components of a still larger system of models for different aspects of life. In adulthood the attachment system operates both self-assertively, to ensure proximity to an identified caregiver, and integrally, to coordinate with the mating and caregiving systems to accomplish the set goal of the sexual pair-bonding system (Ainsworth, 1985, 1989). The working model provides cognitive and affective continuity, not only from past to present to future, but between these integrated systems in adulthood. Our representations of childhood attachment figures strongly influence and become inextricably entwined with our experiences and representations of marital partners.

In what we may call the traditional views of the working model, early experiences are embedded in memory in a model of attachment relationships. This model may be more or less permeable to new information, but in any case it has a *continuous and discrete* existence within our minds.

A NEW UNDERSTANDING OF THE ATTACHMENT SYSTEM'S WORKING MODEL

As noted earlier, Bowlby preferred the term "working model" because he felt the word "working" emphasized the always current, active role of the model in contemporary attachment relationships. But we suggest that, in the light of more recent understandings and speculations about the neurobiology of memory, it is the word "model" that is most problematic. The definition of "model" includes, as first meaning, a "representation, usually in miniature, of a thing to be constructed . . . or of an object, etc., that already exists" (*Webster's Encyclopedic Dictionary*, 1988). We note that, based on this definition, the term "representational model" is guilty, at the very least, of redundancy.

To return to the central point, we question to what extent internalized past attachment experiences exist as a discrete and temporally constant model within our mental world. Certainly, as we have seen, the metaphor of a model can be used somewhat successfully to construct hypotheses about the interplay of our working model with our current experiences to yield certain stances toward attachment relationships—stances that encompass cognitive, affective, and behavioral content. But this type of working model presupposes a neurophysiology that is capable of creating and sustaining such an embedded, long-term feature. There is no reason this should present a problem, given traditional understanding of long-term memory and the brain's ability to create, sustain, and reference memories. Compare the formulations of mental models offered by Bowlby (1969/1982) and the neurologist Young (1967). Bowlby (1969/1982, pp. 80, 81) states: "The use to which a model in the brain is put is to transmit, store, and manipulate information that helps in making predictions . . . The more adequate the model, the more accurate its predictions." Young (1964, p. 23) suggests: "An engineer makes a model of the structure he proposes to build, so that he may test it, on a small scale. Similarly the idea of a model in the brain is that it constitutes a toy that is yet a tool, an imitation world, which we can manipulate."

Recent theories have challenged this understanding of

memory and mental models. Gerald Edelman (1987) has proposed a functional neurophysiology that does *not* include memories in the traditional sense. According to Edelman, the brain *does not store memories* but rather *establishes potentials* for rediscovering previous categories in current situations. In Edelman's (p. 270) words, "Recategorical memory is dynamic, transformational, associative, and distributed — its procedures are *representative* of categorizations, but are not necessarily representations."

But what does this mean? And what are the implications for attachment theory?[3] The first and crucial difference is that there is no stored model to be called upon to guide behavior and feelings when faced with new experiences and situations. Under this theory, stored models do not evoke affects and behaviors; rather, the reverse happens. Motoric stimuli, including behaviors and affects, form the basis for *perception and learning.* Through motoric activity we participate in and test new environments; this stimulates a perceptual search for applicable mental categories; these mental categories, once refound, provide the basis for what Modell (1990, p. 64) calls a "*retranscription* of memory in a new context." To the extent that there are mental models, they are constantly recreated as a synthesis of old categories and new experiences. These synthesized models are a characteristic of the present; they are not stored in memory; rather, their *effects* are incorporated as potentials for influencing renewed models in future experiences.

In this theory, the "working model" of attachment becomes, rather, a particular affective category within the memory. To continue from Modell (1990, p. 66): "Affect categories reflect the memory of a unique constellation of experience (whether veridical or not); they can be thought of as units of experience of the past brought into present time." The affective category of attachment is refound when current behaviors or feelings stimulate a perception of continuity with and similarity to past attachment-related experiences.

We believe this conceptualization of working models as affective categories offers several advantages over the "engineering model" of Bowlby (1969/1982) and the "algorithm model" of Main et al. (1985). At the risk of overgeneralization, we attempt a concise comparative summary. In the "traditional" view of working models, early attachment experiences create an internalized model, containing expectations about behaviors and affects associated with attachment relationships. This internalized model has historical continuity and is used by the individual to guide behaviors and affects in new attachment-relevant situations. The model establishes, for the individual, "rules" or procedures for responding to attachment stimuli. The affective content flows from these rules. The working model precedes, and indeed determines, the perception of a current attachment-relevant experience. One is left making something of a leap from application of the model in respect to a complementary relationship (i.e., infant–parent) to application of the model in respect to a reciprocal relationship (i.e., peer partner). A fixed model does not lend itself readily to the adaptability that is characteristic of normal development. One must appeal to a theory such as Piaget's (1954) accommodation versus assimilation to incorporate adaptability and change of the working model into this view.

In the "new" view of working models proposed here, behaviors and affects that were once associated with attachment form the basis for the perception of potential recategorization of experiences to include both old and new attachment-relevant information. There is no discrete model maintained in the memory, but rather a *potential* to reclassify or recategorize past experiences in the light of current experiences. Perception of attachment-related behaviors and affects *precedes* rediscovery or recreation of the affective category derived from attachment experiences. Affects are not merely part of the content of the working model, they are the mechanism for reactivating in the present the category established in the past. Since continuity is not *situational* (i.e., related to specific situations or relationships) but *motoric* (i.e., related to specific actions and feelings), the extension to peer relationships presents no difficulty. Adaptability is the normative state, as past and present experiences are combined into a renewed category.

Working models are dynamic, associative, affective categories that have the potential to be rediscovered and reformed in new situations. The normative experience of adaptability flows easily from this understanding of working models; it is the pathological experience of nonadaptability or rigidity that needs to be accounted for.

To the extent that projective identification is ubiquitous, many if not all of us, who otherwise are secure in our relationships, have transient periods in which strong negative feelings are projected into our current attachment figures. Insecurely attached individuals manifest this difficulty to a much more obvious degree in regulating their affective processes (Kobak & Sceery, 1988). Unable to view the self as deserving or others as welcoming, the insecurely attached individual is vulnerable to increasingly intense affective distress. Once these strong feeling states are projected onto current relationships, they have the very great likelihood of evoking corresponding feelings in the other individual, which in turn creates a representational identity between past and present attachment experiences. In this self-fulfilling way, further disappointment and frustration in achieving felt security accrue. These attachment experiences are then reinternalized and consolidate constricted attachment patterns.

Israel Rosenfield (1992, pp. 134–135), in discussing the effects of trauma, states:

> We understand the present through the past, an understanding that revises, alters, and reworks the very nature of the past in an ongoing, dynamic process. Psychological or physical trauma appears to "fix" memories. . . . That is, the brain isolates painful experiences and removes them from the dynamic process of understanding. What is fixed is not a "memory" but an organizational ability; and what is abnormal is that this breaks the continuity — the dynamic relation with ongoing experience. . . . The brain cannot block out the pain associated with a given experience without altering its response to other stimuli as well. . . . The brain's organizational abilities normally evolve continuously; organizational patterns that are a consequence of trauma become isolated.

Isolated rigidity is the essence of the organizational patterns of insecure attachment (Bowlby, 1977; Main et al., 1985; West & Sheldon, 1988), which we discuss in the next chapter.

FIVE
PATTERNS OF INSECURE ATTACHMENT

We have discussed the organizing effect of the quality of caregiver responsiveness upon the child's representation of attachment, emphasizing the theory that the persistence of early representations into adulthood depends upon their being confirmed by subsequent attachment events. Having thus been especially strengthened, such working models exert strong selective pressures on latter attachment experiences. In a cyclical and mutually reinforcing way, external events and inner representations are fashioned into attachment patterns. It is these patterns that have attracted the attention of attachment theorists, who are trying to understand both their origins and their effects upon the capacity to form and sustain affectional ties. In the particularly complex task of seeking to understand the insecurely attached individual, the clinician can be guided by discerning how the individual's relational strategies are dominated by set, clearly repetitive patterns of attachment—for this is the essence of insecure attachment.

There exists an extensive body of research on patterns of attachment in infants and young children, but it is not our purpose here to review this research.[1] We shall concentrate upon the patterns of insecure attachment in adults. First, we discuss *feared loss of the attachment relationship* as the pivotal concept in theoretical and clinical understandings of patterns of insecure attachment in adults. Second, we discuss the primary patterns that have been proposed theoretically and empirically. In the next chapter, we will complete the delineation of insecure attachment with a consideration of the attachment theory of defensive processes. That this chapter is devoted more to insecure attachment than to secure attachment should not be taken as indicative of an imbalance in attachment theory. The discussion of secure attachment follows readily from the delineation of the concepts that underpin insecure attachment.

THE FEARED LOSS DYNAMIC

In "Inhibitions, Symptoms, and Anxiety" (1926), Freud placed *loss* at the center of his revised theory of anxiety: Anxiety "can be reduced to a single condition, namely, that of missing someone who is loved and longed for . . . *anxiety appears as a reaction to the felt loss of the object*" (p. 136; emphasis added). Although Freud never abandoned the energic model, the psychology of meaningful interpersonal connections increasingly became the focus of personality study. For example, two of the four danger situations formulated by Freud in 1926 relate directly to object relations: fear of loss of the object and fear of loss of the object's love. In his later works, Freud (1933, 1940) showed a growing recognition of the important role of the early mother–child bond for the later object relations of individuals. Psychoanalysis now concerned itself more with the individual's creation of an interpersonal reality based on actual experiences with significant others. This initiative in psychoanalytic theory reached its fullest expression in the work of theorists such as Sullivan (1953), with his emphasis on the interpersonal field; Fairbairn (1952), who developed object relations theory; and Winnicott (1965), who emphasized the importance of the mother's reflective role in establishing a secure sense of self in the child.

As we have seen, the operation of the attachment system, in conjunction with the complementary response system of the caregiver, creates a template for all future relationships. One theme in Bowlby's theory or story line of attachment comes through strongly: The child is more or less hurt by the responsiveness failures of its caregiver. Things do not go well either in childhood or in later life when this basic parental provision is lacking or compromised. Subsequent relational efforts are hampered by an internal model dominated by feared loss of both the current attachment relationship and of the security that is tied to that relationship. As *felt loss* causes anxiety in Freud's model, so *feared loss* is the central dynamic of insecure adult attachment.

Drawing on material from our research program (see Chapter 7 for a more complete description), we can illustrate the concrete reality of such feared loss. Working with a sample of volunteers drawn from the community, we conducted interviews that included both a projective technique and a semistructured interview component focusing on experiences, behaviors, thoughts, and feelings within reciprocal attachment relationships.

Using the idea of internalized models as individualized attachment stories, we developed a projective technique for investigating the characteristics of an adult's internalized model of attachment. As described in Chapter 7, the technique is based on a set of pictures that depicts attachment-relevant situations with minimal affective clues. Subjects are asked to tell a story about each picture. The underlying rationale, in brief, is that such stories, derived from an indeterminant attachment stimulus, will reflect each individual's internalized attachment model.

The stories our subjects told about the bedtime scene picture illustrated in Figure 5.1 suggest pronounced differences in internal representations of the responsiveness of an attachment figure and the security of an attachment relationship:

"Oh this looks like a scary, scary, nighttime bad dream or nightmare. Or it could be a child saying goodnight to it's mother, but it looks more like the child has woken up and has been frightened and she has come to comfort him and settle him back down again and I feel it will end happily with him feeling calm and going back to sleep."

"Well, I thought of obviously sickness because the child has been sick and, the mother is there, right, to, um . . . obviously . . . uh . . . uh . . . answer his needs and after . . . um . . . I don't know, some type of independence with the child, either he can go back to sleep on his own or take care of his own needs."

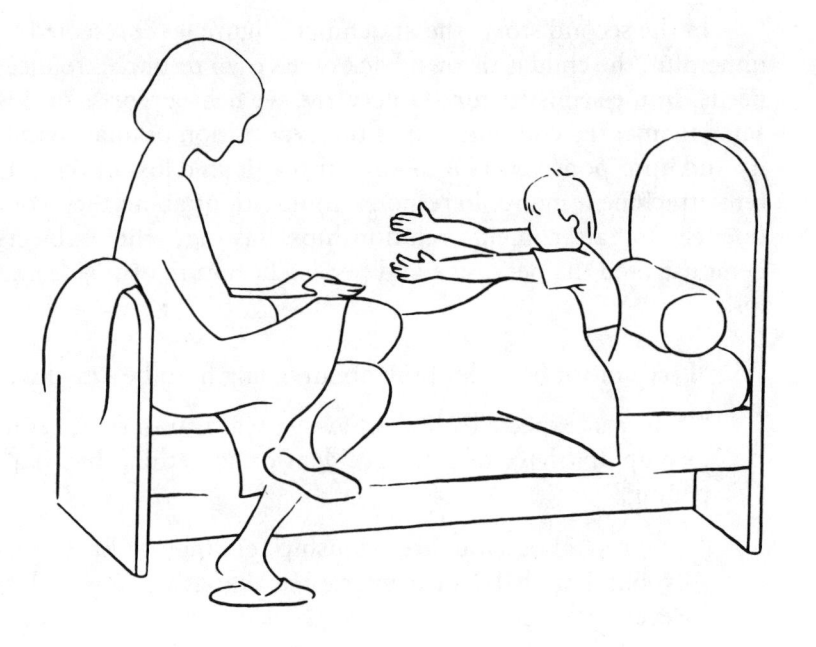

FIGURE 5.1. Bedtime scene.

Each response has a distinctive perceptual and interpretive style. In our formulation, attachment experiences give rise to working models; working models strongly influence the perception and interpretation of any attachment-relevant material and thus underlie the perceptual styles observed in our subjects' responses to the pictures.

For example, both stories contain attachment-eliciting events and feelings on the part of the child ("bad dream or nightmare," "sickness"). The congruency of the parent's responsiveness to the expressed needs of the child, however, varies among the stories. In the first story, the responsiveness of the caregiver ("comfort him") reestablishes felt security in the child. In the second story, the child's attachment behaviors fail to gain comfort and support from the caregiver ("take care of his own needs"). We suggest that these markedly different responses to the same stimulus are isomorphic to our subjects' different working models of attachment.

In the second story, the attachment figure is represented as unhelpful; the child is thrown back on its own resources to meet needs. In the semistructured interview, we hear a reprise of this same theme: the continuation of the expectation of unavailability and unresponsiveness into unremitting feared loss of the current attachment figure. In response to questions about their confidence in attachment relationships lasting, the subjects demonstrated the pervasive and persistent nature of this feared loss:

"I try not to, but I do think about losing him; he's my life."

"If she's unexpectedly late, I have a great fear of that; I conjure up an image of a car accident or something bad happening."

"I worry about our relationship ending; I know it's silly but I wish I had a guarantee that it's going to last forever."

"Logically, I'm confident, but I keep getting these thoughts that he doesn't really love me."

"Over and over the thought crops up in my head that she's going to leave."

The specific and accurate representation arising from repeated experiences of the caregiver's responsiveness failures becomes a generalized working model in which all other persons are perceived as unresponsive. The working model predicts that attachment needs will be unmet, existing attachment figures will be unresponsive and unavailable, and security will be lost and never restored. Instead of having a sustained confidence in the future of the relationship, the insecurely attached individual lives "in constant anxiety lest he lose his attachment figure" (Bowlby, 1977, p. 207).

Our internal representation of the attachment figure has a life of its own that supersedes and usually outlasts the original external other. Because we live simultaneously in an internal and an external reality, we cannot ever lose someone we love. But, paradoxically, because representations "live" in our minds independently of external reality, we *can* experience constant fear of the loss we cannot really encompass. Our internal representations may be constantly threatening withdrawal, disapproval, and displeasure. The cast of characters in such an individual's attachment story share the remembered and predicted traits of unresponsiveness and unavailability.

As we discussed in Chapter 3, attitudes and expectations about attachment that are carried forward to adulthood are *not* the result of working models laid done once and for all in early attachment experiences. Instead, beliefs about attachment that persist have been given special pressure for continuity through having been confirmed by subsequent events, making them more powerful and entrenching them as organizers of later attachment relationships. And once they are projected onto new relationships, further disappointment and frustration of attachment desires are likely to accrue. These attachment experiences are then reinternalized and consolidate constricted relational styles. Faithful adherence to a style of relating is striking even though it often prevents the individual from finding and accepting satisfactory relationships; self-sabotaging interactions and painful feelings are recreated over and over. There is a bondage to a mode of relating learned originally within the family that narrows the possibilities for establishing ties to others.

Patterns of insecure attachment develop in order to prevent the individual from reexperiencing a situation of frustration and helplessness that previously caused severe anxiety and sadness. The individual seeks, in other words, to avoid the recurrence of an unbearable threat: threat of the loss of the current attachment relationship. Such clearly defensive patterns may have enabled individuals to offset deficient childhood attachment environments and to lead reasonably satisfactory lives. In this regard, Cassidy and Kobak (1987) point out that the avoidant response in children is adaptive in the sense of being a solution that minimizes the child's attachment behaviors, which are likely to result in the caregiver's angry rejection, while at the same time allowing the child to maintain some degree of physical proximity to the caregiver. Perhaps, in this context, it is difficult to decide whether an attachment pattern is basically adaptive or defensive, that is, adaptive in protecting the child against further experiences of painful rebuff. As clinicians, we are likely to see such people as adults after their lifelong attachment pattern has been threatened or undermined by a quantitative or qualitative increase in closeness. For these individuals, the possibility of an intimate relationship, although frequently desired, shatters their detachment so that feelings become intense.

Working out the most commonly observed patterns has been one of the most pertinent contributions of attachment theory and research. Before describing these patterns, we should first like to point out that they are comprised of attitudes toward and expectations about attachment of which the individual may be more or less unaware. Just as the psychoanalytic concepts of character, protective organization, and neurotic styles have not been seen as typically conscious, so we have to allow that patterns of attachment may be practised wholly outside of awareness. They are part of an individual's unwitting efforts to adapt to his or her attachment relationships within the framework of his or her working model and to contain the conflicts that they evoke.

PATTERNS OF INSECURE ATTACHMENT

We shall begin with Bowlby's descriptive scheme of patterns of insecure attachment behavior, with a view to examining how each pattern arises, how it works, and what defensive purposes it serves. We next describe three patterns of insecure attachment that have been validated conceptually and empirically against Ainsworth's patterns of attachment in infancy (Main, 1991). It will become plain to the reader from the description that follows that the various forms of insecure attachment move from the more detached, distant patterns to the close, enmeshed ones.

Compulsive Self-Sufficiency

Individuals whom Bowlby has described as compulsively self-sufficient deny their need for a loving close relationship to anyone and give self-sufficiency a central place in conducting their lives. The giving up of meaningful contact with others and the loss of recognition of their true feelings is often massive. Their self-sufficiency tends to irradiate to all areas of their relationships to other people. As Bowlby (1977, p. 207) observes, "So far from seeking the love and care of others, an individual who exhibits this pattern insists on keeping a stiff upper lip and doing everything for himself whatever the conditions." The defensive flavor of this apparent "switching off" of attachment feelings is obvious. The chronic inability to feel close to anyone, masquerading as self-sufficiency, leads to perpetual feelings of loneliness and yearnings for support. Yet any deep attachment threatens to revive past memories of old deprivations and hurts and produces withdrawal.

In the prototype for development of compulsive self-sufficiency, the activation of the attachment system in infancy and childhood is not met with appropriate responses and therefore is never successfully terminated. Attachment behaviors (e.g., crying, clinging) do not evoke a comforting response from and increased proximity to the caregiver, but rather provoke displeasure and rejection by the caregiver. As the child's distress increases, the attachment behaviors become more pronounced and demanding. This simply provokes more pronounced rejection. Through repeated similar experiences, the child learns that attachment behaviors lead to rejection and are therefore dangerous. The system is eventually deactivated completely by "the defensive exclusion . . . of sensory inflow of any and every kind that might activate attachment behavior and feeling" (Bowlby, 1980, p. 70). Main (1981) argued that deactivation of attachment behaviors offers, in these circumstances, the best possibility for achieving the system's set goal of proximity to the caregiver: The caregiver rejects the demanding child but is willing to maintain proximity as long as the child is undemanding.

Compulsive self-sufficiency thus originates with cumulative and persistent failures in the caregiver holding environment (Winnicott, 1965). Caregivers who are woefully deficient in empathy or who never understand why the child cries or who push the child away are examples of parental holding failures. The child's reaction to this loss of the caregiver as a responsive and protective figure is withdrawal into a kind of self-holding (Modell,

1984). As Guntrip (1969, p. 24) notes in reference to the child-hood experiences of schizoid individuals, "When you cannot get what you want from the person you need," you (the child) are forced to be all-sufficient within yourself. This solution, clearly adaptive in the face of significant failures of caregiver holding, later becomes the "symptom" of what we refer to as a dysfunctional pattern of attachment.

Compulsive Care Giving

There is a pattern very similar to compulsive self-sufficiency, one in which the individual is always in the giving role, never allowing himself or herself to receive care. Although Bowlby does not explicate the antecedents of compulsive care giving as precisely as he does those for compulsive self-sufficiency, the general developmental pathway is clear. As Bowlby (1977, p. 207) states, "The typical childhood experience of such people is to have a mother who, due to depression or some other disability, was unable to care for the child but, instead, welcomed being cared for and perhaps also demanded help in caring for younger siblings." This description of the experiential antecedents of compulsive care giving suggests that it is likely that the activation of the child's attachment system evoked anxious and ineffective concern, rather than comforting responsiveness, from the parent. Through repeated experiences, the child has learned that attachment behaviors provoke distress in the parent. Consequently, conflict is experienced whenever the child's attachment system is activated. A solution is sought that will maintain the child's relational proximity to the parent. The care-giving response is such a solution because it suppresses the child's own attachment behaviors while at the same time allowing for proximity to the parent. The parent's distress elicits the child's care giving, setting the stage, as it were, for an association between attachment and care giving within the child's working model of attachment.

As a result of these experiences with the parent, the child has learned that a relationship can only be attained by accepting the parent's definition of the grounds for attachment. To achieve relational proximity, the child has no choice but to submit to this definition. Paradoxically, then, proximity to the parent is gained at the cost of the child's attachment behaviors; that is, deactivation of the child's attachment system offers, in these circumstances, the best chance to achieve a degree of proximity to the parent. The child's need for care is renounced for the sake of maintaining proximity to the parent.

The limitless quality of the parent's neediness, coupled with the frustration experienced in the face of felt and expressed needs, also teaches the child to fear neediness as inevitable weakness and loss of control. The child has learned that to feel or express neediness is a threat to well-being and security. In the case of Mary, described in Chapter 2, any strong attachment desire evoked intense anxiety. The desire was experienced as weakening her, making her fear that its expression would leave her helpless and out of control like her mother. Thus, she played the role of caregiver in which she administered to the needfulness of the other person. The role of caregiver, although it meant denial and frustration of her attachment desires, removed her from the more feared reality of helplessness and lack of control. Being in control is reflected in the "passive into active" defensive strategy of compulsive care giving that enables the individual to be an active initiator rather than, as was the case in childhood, a helpless victim of attachment.

It is important to differentiate this kind of care giving from care-giving initiatives that arise properly later in life in reciprocal relationships and true parental relationships. These adult care-giving behaviors arise from the care-giving system, and are complementary to the attachment system. In contrast, caretaking behaviors directed from a child to a parent arise from the child's attachment system and lead to dysfunctional relationships later in life as the individual loses any ability to express need or ask for care, yet retains a pervasive, unsatisfied neediness and longing for care. For such an individual in adulthood, the attachment and care-giving systems do not balance each other to yield stable reciprocal relationships but rather reinforce patterns of exclusive care giving and the suppression of care seeking.

Anxious Attachment

In "The Making and Breaking of Affectional Bonds" (1977), Bowlby outlines how individuals establish attachment patterns in response to the ways in which their parents have related to them. In terms of the caregiver's responsiveness, the childhood experiences of those individuals Bowlby has described as anxiously attached are "experiences that shake a person's confidence that his attachment figure will be available to him when desired" (p. 213). This description could be readily applied to the experiential antecedents of compulsive self-reliant individuals. But, in describing the conditions predisposing an individual to anxious attachment, Bowlby emphasizes *interruptions of care,* in particular interruptions of the primary attachment relationship, substitute care that fails to provide one primary caregiver, and threatened interruptions caused by the caregiver's actions (e.g., suicidal gestures or threats to abandon the child or send the child away if he or she is bad). Clearly, it is the confusing and contradictory nature of the attachment experiences that differentiates these experiences from those predisposing an individual to compulsive self-sufficiency. The individual who exhibits compulsive self-sufficiency experienced consistency: Whenever attachment behaviors were expressed, the result was rejection. The individual who exhibits anxious attachment experienced inconsistency, either through changing external circumstances or through the inconsistent responsiveness of the caregiver. The caregiver would sometimes be responsive, sometimes rejecting, sometimes anxious — seemingly, to the young child, capriciously and unpredictably. The child learns that no pattern of response can be automatically assumed but that activation of attachment must always include watchfulness and uncertainty. In another context, Dorothy Sayers (1987, p. 17) has spoken of the consequences of such a perception. If the attachment figure's reactions "are conceived as being arbitrary, capricious and irrational, we shall continue in a state of terror and bewilderment, since we shall never know from one minute to the next what we are expected to be doing, or why, or what we have to expect."

Attachment theory teaches us that proximity-seeking in childhood is a means of establishing security with the caregiver. Anxious attachment, as the term denotes, fails to achieve the function of attachment. Because security has not been experienced, proximity-seeking tends to be treated as a goal in its own right. In the adult, although a close personal relationship may be maintained or desired, this relationship does not contribute to security, but more often exacerbates insecurity. In this case, the associated fear is not of the loss of security because there is no real security provided by the relationship. Rather, feared loss becomes feared loss of proximity to the attachment figure. Or, to put it another way, in the continued absence of security, the original function of attachment is "forgotten"; the function becomes instead congruent with the means intended to achieve security. The goal, therefore, in anxious attachment, becomes the maintenance of proximity to an attachment figure; the fear becomes loss of or separation from that individual.

A response like that of Joan described in Chapter 2 is dramatically illustrative of anxious attachment. Joan appears to have clung to the belief that so long as she was able to maintain proximity to her husband the dangers of living would not affect her. The only danger she feared was separation from her husband.

Main's Patterns of Insecure Attachment

Mary Main and her colleagues developed the Adult Attachment Interview (AAI) to assess the patterns of attachment in the adult. To summarize this assessment strategy: Within the interview, the coherency of discourse about past attachment-relevant experiences, particularly with parents, is subjected to detailed semantic analysis. In this context, coherency has a particular meaning and refers to the maxims of coherent discourse as explicated by Grice (1975). The coherency of discourse is taken to be a direct reflection of the adult's "current state of mind with respect to attachment," which is Main's formulation for the working model. A judgment of coherent discourse leads to a classification of autonomous (secure) attachment; incoherent discourse is analyzed for the type and context of incoherences to assign one of three categories of insecure attachment.

"Dismissing" adults (cf. Bowlby's compulsive self-sufficiency [1980] and Ainsworth's avoidant pattern for infants [Ainsworth et al., 1978]) are characterized by a cognitive organization of attachment-relevant information based on denial of the occurrence, importance, or effects of attachment relationships. Rosenstein, Horowitz, Steidl, and Oreston (1992, p. 497) have summarized the state of mind with regard to attachment of dismissing individuals as follows:

> There is an idealization of the parents or portrayal of negative experiences with the parents as normal. Frequently, these individuals lack memory for childhood, or, if negative memories do occur, they regard themselves as unaffected by them. Often, they highly value achievement, self-reliance, personal strength, or cunning. These qualities are sometimes cited as rationalizations for the lack of effect on self of negative experiences. . . . These individuals are the least likely of any attachment groups to avow internal distress. However, others view them as hostile and provocative, [prone] to act out their all-too-obvious inner disharmony and affective dysregulation.

The second major pattern of insecure attachment classified by the AAI is "preoccupied" (cf. Ainsworth's [1978] ambivalent pattern for infants). Individuals classified as preoccupied cannot free themselves from a preoccupying enmeshment with past attachment relationships. This enmeshment may be accompanied by *intensely angry affect* that seemingly overwhelms the individual inappropriately and consistently in attempts to discuss the attachment figure or attachment-related events. Conversely, the enmeshment can be expressed as a *passively quiet, somewhat distracted continuing involvement* with attachment events or attachment figures, such that there is an almost complete failure of perspective-taking. Both the angry and the passive preoccupied styles, but particularly the latter, seem conceptually related to problems of ego boundaries.

The third major pattern is a superordinate pattern that may occur in conjunction with either insecure pattern or with a pattern of secure attachment. This is the pattern of unresolved/disorganized responses to loss (cf. Main & Solomon's [1986] disorganized patterns in infants). Typically, this pattern occurs as a sequelae to actual loss of an attachment figure, through death or permanent separation, though other conditions that may lead to a state of mind classified as unresolved/disorganized are being investigated (Kenneth Adam, personal communication, May 14, 1992). Individuals classified as unresolved exhibit a variety of cognitive disturbances in attempting to discuss an attachment-relevant loss and have seemingly failed to assimilate this loss and move beyond it. Because the effect may be quite circumscribed, individuals who are classified as unresolved/disorganized are always given an accompanying classification of autonomous (secure), dismissing (avoidant), or preoccupied (enmeshed/ambivalent).

INSECURE ATTACHMENT
AS INCOMPLETE MOURNING

Although Main (1991) restricts the classification of unresolved/disorganized reaction to loss to a particular set of circumstances and cognitive indices, one can relate characteristics of Main's patterns of dismissing and preoccupied attachment as well as characteristics of Bowlby's patterns of insecure attachment to variations of an incomplete mourning reaction. Loss in which an attachment bond is broken irrevocably sets in process the experience of mourning (Bowlby, 1963). As we pointed out in Chapter 3, chronic experiences of parental unresponsiveness, rebuff, or gross inconsistency can summate and have all the emotional impact of a complete loss. From the point of view of pathological mourning, the single most important cause of insecure attachment lies in the individual's inability to master the loss of a longed for but never fully experienced tender relationship to the caregiver. Unresolved mourning is always associated with the giving up of authentic relatedness to others and a relative detachment from one's true feelings.

In the compulsive self-reliant/dismissing pattern, the detachment and withdrawal are of a much greater magnitude than in the case of the anxious/preoccupied pattern. The turning away from intimate personal relationships is pervasive. As Bowlby (1977, p. 207) observed of the compulsive self-reliant individual: "So far from seeking the love and care of others, a person who exhibits this pattern insists on keeping a stiff upper lip and doing everything for himself whatever the conditions." The self-sufficiency is in many ways a pseudo self-sufficiency that covers a soft-hearted center full of perpetual feelings of loneliness and unexpressed yearning for love and support.

Main's (1985) characterization of dismissing individuals provides the best and most obvious explanation of their withdrawal from meaningful contacts with other persons. Specifically, the idealized versions given by these individuals of their childhood attachment experiences bespeaks repressed feelings of denial of loss. The inability of dismissing individuals to face the feelings of anger and sadness that accompany disappointments in the relationship with their parents suggests that grief has only been experienced in part, and loss only partially admitted. As has often been observed, this inability to recognize and express anger and sadness leads to the inability to feel and express attachment emotions. The dismissing individual's detachment from any kind of deep feeling is general and pervading.

In the case of the anxious/preoccupied patterns, the individual seems not to believe that it is obligatory to say good-bye to a "lost" attachment relationship. Rather, there is a persistent effort to recover this lost relationship, often accompanied by intense anger and reproach expressed toward the parent. (As we noted earlier, the relationship can be "lost" in terms of the ability to provide security even in the absence of actual loss.) The inability to break free from an enmeshed dependency on an ambivalently regarded parent necessarily compromises the individual's ability to form authentic ties to new attachment figures.

SECURE ATTACHMENT

Over the course of development, the seeking of felt security leads to discovering how responsive the attachment environment is to our needs. If all goes well and we receive love and comfort, it also leads to feelings of being worthy of care and to the ability to get others to give us the care we need. This outcome shows most clearly in the level of confidence we have that our current attachment relationships will provide needed security.

There is an old saying that "The proof of the pudding is in the eating." It can be paraphrased for attachment: The proof of attachment is in the feared loss of the security achieved through the relationship. It should be recognized that in the above sentence the phrase is *not* feared loss of the *relationship,* but rather feared loss of the *security* invested in the relationship. Because security is achieved through the attachment relationship, there is a component of feared loss even in secure relationships. But in secure relationships the fear is understood as a necessary consequence of the investment of security in another person, is accepted as an affect appropriate to the relationship, and is kept in bounds by the presence of a confident belief in the attachment figure's reliable availability. As Guntrip (1969, p. 21) has put it in another context, "In the case of a continuing good object relationship of major importance such as with a parent or marriage partner, we have . . . confidence in the continuing possession of the good object in an externally real sense in the present and the future."

Main's Pattern of Autonomy

John Bowlby did not define secure attachment *as a behavioral pattern.* Indeed, it is both easier and more sensible to define the patterns of insecurity, which are characterized by set, relatively inflexible, and constricted behaviors and affects. In contrast, the hallmark of secure attachment is freshness of response and freedom from prescribed and proscribed behaviors. Nonetheless, Ainsworth et al. (1978) were able to differentiate secure infants (of the "B" pattern) on the basis of positive indices rather than simply the absence of negative indices. Similarly, Main (1985) has delineated the key characteristics of a pattern of secure attachment which she has designated "autonomous." In the context of the AAI, the autonomous individual exhibits a willingness and ability to cooperate with the interviewer, to recall attachment-related memories and feelings, and to speak of such experiences with consistency and clarity. This collaborative stance results in an interview transcript that is characterized by Main as "highly coherent." In Main's system, a highly coherent transcript is the result of current security about attachment, a security that allows the individual to simultaneously value and maintain both independence and connectedness.

Theoretical Distinctions

Secure attachment is differentiated from insecure attachment by the *higher* threshold for the activation of the attachment system, and the greater ability to maintain or reestablish the felt security that signals termination of attachment behaviors. Because the securely attached adult's sense of subjective confidence in the security of the attachment relationship is quite high, the number and type of situations that evoke attachment behaviors are relatively few. Absences or separations of a few days, for example, are well tolerated. In an essential way, the securely attached individual's sense of a secure base is demonstrated in the absence of the attachment figure. As the maintenance of proximity to the attachment figure becomes an internalized representational process, separations (actual or anticipated) are increasingly well tolerated and do not lead to the suppression of exploratory and coping behaviors that characterizes activation of attachment behaviors. The exclusive predominance of attachment behaviors in the secure adult are only likely to be shown under severe or prolonged distress.

In adults, as Bretherton (1985, p. 12) points out, "The waning of attachment behaviors does not, however, imply the waning of the attachment system." The way to understand this, we suggest, is to put the accent not on frequency, but on intensity. For securely attached adults, coping responses such as talking about problems, seeking to understand the meaning of stressful events, and other cognitive strategies that reduce anxiety and lead to effective coping, mean that most difficulties of daily living can be successfully overcome. Only in situations of severe distress, such as illness, physical injury, or emotional upset, is the attachment system activated with near similar intensity to that seen in children.

This way of looking at attachment behavior in adults suggests that the various responses to stressful situations can be arranged in hierarchical fashion. The attachment system can be activated at various levels of intensity, determined by the degree of perceived threat, and correlated with the strength of the need for proximity to the attachment figure. For the securely attached adult, low to moderate levels of activation, as result from the ordinary exigencies of daily life, lead to the use of cognitive strategies (i.e., reliance on working models of the attachment figure and the security of the relationship) to maintain "proximity." The sense of threat is diminished and the sense of security maintained not by seeking physical proximity to the attachment figure (as is true of the anxiously attached person), but by reference to the working model of the attachment figure. Only when the stressors are extraordinary is the activation of the attachment system strong enough to require physical proximity to the attachment figure and to overwhelm other behavioral systems. In contrast, the insecurely attached adult has an internal working model that does not allow the successful use of cognitive strategies for meeting attachment needs. Thus the insecurely attached adult will have a lower threshold for expression of concrete attachment behaviors and will not be able to easily reestablish a sense of security. Because activation of the attachment system suppresses other behavioral systems, coping responses connected with other behavioral systems will not be as readily available.

Use of the Attachment Figure

The securely attached adult can acknowledge felt distress in a modulated way and turn to supportive and trusted relationships for comfort. Particularly during periods of emotional upset, comfort often needs to be expressed in concrete attachment behaviors that reassure the individual. Put simply, felt security at these times has a lot to do with having someone available who will respond to our feelings and even take supportive action. The special warmth that often accompanies attachment comes just from these tangible reassurances that one is understood. Further, in extreme life crises such as bereavement, illness, or physical injury to oneself or a dependent child, attachment behaviors take a highly prototypical form, including the wish to be held, the freedom to cry, and the predominance over other behavioral systems.

One of the primary behavioral consequences of insecure attachment is an inability to use attachment figures effectively to reestablish threatened or lost security. In the next chapter we reexamine the historical use of defensive processes to try to characterize the mechanisms underlying this inability.

S I X

DEFENSIVE PROCESSES
IN ATTACHMENT THEORY

I n preceding chapters we discussed the developmental antecedents and prototypical styles of relating that characterize patterns of insecure attachment. In this chapter we tackle the more theoretical issue of a formulation of patterns of insecure attachment as *defensive processes*. Bowlby (1980) framed defensive processes in the language of information processing; later attachment writers also continue to explain the patterns of insecure attachment as arising from deficits or disturbances in the processing of attachment-relevant information. Just as *repression* is the key to understanding the psychoanalytic theory of defense, so *defensive exclusion* is the key to understanding the attachment theory of defense.

In a chapter entitled, "An Information Processing Approach to Defense," Bowlby (1980) refers to studies in neurophysiology, cognitive psychology, and human information processing as the basis for his theory of defensive structures. In general he uses these studies to support four propositions:

1. "Sensory inflow," whether coming from the external or the internal environment, is subject to "central control" such that it "goes through many stages of selection, interpretation and appraisal before it can have any influence on behaviour" (pp. 44–45).
2. Most sensory inflow is "routinely excluded from further processing in order that [the individual's] capacities are not overloaded. . . . Most selective exclusion, therefore, is both necessary and adaptive" (p. 45).

3. Only the final stage of processing is at the conscious level. Up to then, any "sensory inflow can be processed outside awareness and . . . further inflow can either be enhanced or reduced" (p. 52).
4. "Consciousness can be regarded as a state of mental structures that greatly facilitates certain distinctive types of processing to occur" (p. 54).

With reference to the last point, Bowlby includes in the role of consciousness the ordering of processed information, the retrieval of old information from long-term memory, the comparison of different kinds of information, decision making based on evaluation of information, and "the inspection of certain overlearned and automated action systems, together with the representational models linked to them, that may be proving maladapted" (p. 54).

Selective exclusion, then, is an adaptive mechanism for ensuring that relevant data is attended to in preference to irrelevant data. Selective exclusion differentiates information from data, or signal from noise. We all know the common experience of a parent who is preoccupied with a task at hand: the noise of his children playing is easily ignored (i.e., selectively excluded), but the sound of his child's crying captures the parent's attention immediately.

Defensive exclusion, by contrast, is the persistent exclusion of some particular data that should be attended to as information or signal but instead is treated as noise because past experiences have led to suffering or pain when the information is fully processed (Peterfreund, 1971). According to attachment theory, information is excluded from awareness to serve some need —usually a rather intense need—of the individual to resolve a conflict, to reduce anxiety, or to remove a sense of threat to the security of the individual. The defensive exclusion of information, like its psychoanalytic conceptual counterpart, repression, can thus be an adaptive stratagem—adaptive, however, only in some limited way, for the ability to integrate information relevant to attachment is a hallmark of secure attachment. Defensive exclusion is a response to a threat; it occurs because past experiences have led to suffering and pain when the information was fully processed.

Defensive exclusion can occur at one of two general levels: *Perceptual exclusion* leads to the deactivation of the attachment system, and *preconscious exclusion* leads to stopping the processing of information prior to the conscious level, and thus to the "cognitive disconnection of a response from the interpersonal situation that elicited it" (Bowlby, 1980, p. 67). These two processes of exclusion form the basis for differentiating maladaptive patterns of attachment. Bowlby subsumes all other defenses (e.g., projection, idealization, conversion, displacement, and the like) under the general headings of defensive beliefs and defensive activities, which assist exclusions by directing attention away from the information being excluded. Underlying each of Bowlby's patterns of insecure attachment is a hypothesized, particular type of persistent defensive exclusion of some data that is treated as noise rather than information.

PERCEPTUAL EXCLUSION: DEACTIVATION OF ATTACHMENT

Defensive exclusion is easily translated into the pattern of behavioral consequences that Bowlby called compulsive self-sufficiency. As we discussed earlier, Bowlby sees this pattern as evolving from experiences that were rejecting of attachment and that therefore led the individual to "deactivate" the attachment system by excluding from processing any signals for activation. Cassidy and Kobak (1987) have extended Bowlby's conception into consequences for affect regulation and working models. They suggest that the masking of negative affect serves the same function as avoidance of attachment behaviors; that is, it keeps the caregiver close by avoiding stimuli that have caused rejection and distancing. With development, the necessity to mask negative affect generalizes to a "defensive restriction in affective expression" which is interpreted by others as meaning that the individual is unaffected by others. The interpersonal behavioral consequences of this stance is to decrease the likelihood that others will attempt to engage the individual in emotional or affective interactions. The working model that others form of the individual thus serves to complement the individual's need to avoid activation of the attachment system.

Cassidy and Kobak further hypothesize that the individual's working model includes views of relationships that deemphasize the importance of giving and receiving care, and information-processing biases that function to control or deny affective distress. They use idealization as an example of such a bias: The individual constructs an idealized semantic (i.e., general) model of parents, self, and their relationship that contradicts and denies the real episodic (i.e., specific) model based on actual experiences (cf. Tulving, 1972). The consequence of defensive restriction in affective expression and of this type of working model is to maintain the pattern of defensively excluding information that would activate the attachment system; hence, a pattern of compulsive self-sufficiency is established and continued.

One problem with this model of deactivation of the attachment system is that it implies that the system ceases to function and is, in fact, permanently "turned off." This could be interpreted as implying that in normal circumstances the system operates intermittently, turning on and off in response to activation signals. Bretherton (1985) has proposed that to fulfill its function of ensuring safety, the attachment system cannot be merely intermittently active: It must be continually active, monitoring the environment to assess proximity to the caregiver and the familiarity of the surroundings. For this reason, one must recognize that *attachment behaviors* are only intermittently activated; the *attachment system* itself, however, is continually active as an environmental monitor.

Is the attachment system deactivated as a monitor, or is it just attachment behaviors that are deactivated in the case of compulsive self-sufficiency? Bowlby believes that it is the system itself that is deactivated. Other authors (e.g., Main, 1981; Cassidy & Kobak, 1987; Bretherton, 1985) hypothesize that the system remains active, both in terms of its environmental monitoring activity and in terms of orientation to achieving a set goal.

Do different answers to the above question make any difference? The answer cannot be anything but yes. If the attachment system is completely deactivated, then by definition all attachment-relevant information is excluded from processing and therefore cannot influence behavior. If the attachment system remains active as a monitor, then attachment-relevant information is processed and does influence behavior (and affect), albeit according to a working model that mitigates against the expression of any attachment behaviors or affects.

As we have seen, Bowlby presents compulsive self-sufficiency as the result of the defensive exclusion of attachment-relevant information *at the initial perceptual level:* The information is never allowed into the processing system. But there is a logical inconsistency to this view. If attachment-relevant information is completely excluded and does not affect behaviors, then behaviors should be *random* in relation to attachment. To believe that behaviors are *patterned* in relation to attachment necessitates the corollary belief that attachment-relevant information is recognized and processed and used to determine behavioral responses. The behavioral response of choice may be complete avoidance and the *appearance* of defensive exclusion, but the consistency of the response betrays the careful attendance to attachment-relevant information. Therefore, we believe that it makes more sense to model compulsive self-sufficiency not as the complete defensive exclusion of attachment-relevant information, but rather as the complete defensive exclusion of attachment behaviors. Compulsive self-sufficiency, under this model, is not the result of an information-processing deficit.

The counterargument could be advanced that the nonrandom response defined by compulsive self-sufficiency is the *absence of attachment behaviors.* This response could evolve under two conditions: The first is the exclusion of any information or stimuli that would evoke an attachment behavior (this is Bowlby's theory); the second is the processing of such information and stimuli according to a working model that leads to the complete suppression of attachment behaviors (this is the alternate theory we ascribe to here). These conditions would be equally probable only if the behaviors under consideration were *unique* to attachment. If such behaviors were present only when attachment needs predominated, then the complete absence of attachment behaviors could not assist us in deciding which condition is more likely to pertain.

But as we noted in Chapter 1, behaviors that are designated attachment behaviors are not unique, in adults, to activation of the attachment system, but rather are connected to multiple behavioral systems. Therefore, the complete suppression of behaviors relevant to attachment would require much more than the defensive exclusion of attachment-relevant information: It would require the exclusion of information relevant to a number of behavioral systems. Unfortunately, the appealing simplicity of the model of defensive exclusion at the perceptual level is at odds with the complexity of the model of interrelated behavioral systems in adults. One or the other has to give way.

Our formulation agrees with the model proposed by Main (1981) under which the suppression of attachment behaviors actually becomes, in a sense, an attachment behavior itself. Given an attachment figure who is made angry and rejecting by the expression of attachment behaviors, then the best way to achieve the set goal of the attachment system (which is, we must remember, proximity to the attachment figure) is to suppress those behaviors. The attachment figure will be more willing to maintain proximity to a quiet, undemanding infant than to a crying, clinging, reaching (all attachment behaviors) infant. So information relevant to attachment is not excluded but rather comes to be associated with distinct behavioral sequelae characterized by the absence of any externally identifiable attachment behavior.

EXCLUSION FROM CONSCIOUSNESS: DISCONNECTION OF CAUSE AND EFFECT

Defensive exclusion of activation signals at the perceptual level is not the only form of defensive exclusion hypothesized by Bowlby. Activation can be allowed but accurate interpretation of the meaning of activation disallowed. Bowlby (1980, p. 65) implies that it is this form of defensive exclusion that is most likely to be supported by defensive activities and beliefs "to divert [the individual's] attention away from whoever, or whatever, may be responsible for his reactions" Bowlby places a lot of emphasis on the defensive activity of giving care to others, with the subsequent development of a stable pattern of compulsive care giving in relationships.

Compulsive Care Giving

As noted in the previous chapter, compulsive care giving probably derives from experiences in which activation of the child's attachment behaviors evokes anxious and ineffective concern, rather than comforting responsiveness, from the caregiver. The child learns that attachment behaviors provoke distress (as opposed to anger and rejection as in the evolution of compulsive self-sufficiency) in the attachment figure.

This model depends on an infant at the opposite end of the perceptual scale from Mahler et al.'s (1975) "autistic" infant who has little or no ability to differentiate environmental components, much less the affective responses of such components. Under this model, compulsive care giving depends on an infant's ability to discriminate relatively fine affective differences in the attachment figure. This ability may not be as improbable as it sounds, given recent research demonstrating the relatively sophisticated perceptual abilities of even very young infants, and the opportunity for the elaboration of such abilities over the course of childhood, as working models (Tronick & Adamson, 1980).

A more serious problem lies in the twist of mind necessary to construe *reinterpretation* of information as *exclusion* of information. In Bowlby's paradigm of defensive processes, it is not attachment relevant information that is excluded in this instance, but rather the *meaning* of this information for activation of attachment behaviors. Care giving is a diversionary behavioral pattern: The river of attachment does not flow freely in a natural channel but rather is dammed and diverted into a neighboring river. The dam is the exclusion; the diversion (into care giving) prevents insupportable pressure on the dam.

The metaphor is fine in a general sense. But to say that a given pattern arises from the misinterpretation of the meaning of activation is to explain nothing because it applies to all patterns of insecure attachment. To return to the metaphor: The fact of misinterpretation is the dam, but that fact does not explain why the diversion into one particular other river rather than another occurs.

Why the diversion to care giving in particular? The care-giving behavioral system is the complement of the infant's attachment system. This system is dormant in infancy and also usually dorment in early childhood, although early intermittent activation can be seen frequently in the protectiveness of older siblings regarding younger siblings. If activation of attachment behaviors provokes distress in the caregiver, then the caregiver's distress could activate the child's care-giving system. The expression of care-giving behaviors on the child's part could then lead to decreased distress of the attachment figure and therefore her increased tolerance for closeness to the attachment-needing child. Using the same model under which anger and rejection in response to the child's attachment behaviors led to suppression of those behaviors in order to enhance the probability of proximity to the attachment figure, the caregiver's distress in response to these behaviors can lead to care-giving behaviors in the child. In these circumstances, an association between attachment and care giving within the child's working model eventuates: The set goal of attachment (proximity to the attachment figure) will be most likely achieved through care-giving behaviors rather than attachment behaviors; care-giving behaviors become associated with activation of attachment needs, and thus a pattern of compulsive care giving develops.

Conceptually, this model is similar to the one proposed by Bowlby, representing more of a shift in emphasis than a shift in content. The emphasis is not on the nature of the exclusion (the "dam") but rather on the nature of the substitutionary behaviors (the alternate "river").

Anxious Attachment

The final pattern of insecure attachment explicated by Bowlby is anxious attachment. The defensive exclusion that Bowlby proposed here is another variety of disconnection of cause and effect. The individual comes to "dwell so insistently on the details of his own reactions and sufferings that he has no time to consider what the interpersonal situation responsible for his reactions may really be" (Bowlby, 1980, p. 65). As noted previously, the antecedent of anxious attachment is inconsistency in responsiveness, either through changing external circumstances or through inconsistent responsiveness of the caregiver. The development of a pattern of anxious attachment from such experiences makes sense. But to categorize this response as a variety of defensive exclusion seems to us to be stretching the point. We return again to the issue of the relative importance of what is being excluded versus the importance of what is being promoted. Under all conditions of insecure attachment, the normal operation of the attachment system is excluded. To differentiate patterns, one must attend to what is substituted to maximize the probability of achieving the set goal of the attachment system.

Attention to substitutionary strategies is perhaps nowhere more evident than in the (AAI) system for classifying patterns of adult attachment behaviors. Of particular interest here is not so much the classifications themselves as the derivation of the classifications. Each classification represents a particular style of thinking, speaking, and feeling in regards to attachment figures and events. The hallmark of secure, autonomous attachment (F) is an unrestricted, free-flowing, collaborative style of discourse. The patterns of insecure attachment (U, Ds, E) are derived by attending to the specific manner in which discourse is restricted, diverted, or uncontrolled.

GENERAL WEAKNESSES OF BOWLBY'S MODEL OF DEFENSIVE EXCLUSION

As we have described above, Bowlby framed his explanation of defensive processes within an information-processing model. The primary mechanism of defense derives from the adaptive mechanism of selective exclusion, which ensures that attention is focused on signal rather than on noise. In defensive exclusion, certain types of signals are habitually ignored.

In explicating behavioral control systems, Bowlby argued directly from available evidence and used a theory that was necessary to, but not analogous to, an explanation of the evidence. By contrast, in explicating defensive processes, Bowlby—like Freud before him—infers a theory for psychology from a popular theory within another branch of scientific enquiry. Schafer (1983) and Kohut (1984) have criticized the psychoanalytic concept of defense for reflecting an archaic mechanistic scientism, based as it is on analogy to the mechanics of energy as understood by nineteenth-century physics. Similarly, Bowlby's model of defensive processes is based on analogy to the mechanics of information processing as understood by early twentieth- century cognitive science. Both Freud and Bowlby locate the defensive process in an individual's intrapsychic "machinery" which operates, according to Freud, by the inexorable laws of nineteenth-centry physics or, according to Bowbly, by the equally fixed rules of early twentieth-century information processing. Bowlby's formulation of defensive processes is overly mechanistic and increasingly out of date: It offers a computerized version of attachment that fails to correspond well with more current neurological research and understandings of the particular constraints on information processing that characterize the human brain (cf. Rosenfield, 1992). It seems unlikely that defensive exclusion is a more *accurate* formulation than repression.

AN ALTERNATIVE APPROACH

Bowlby was keenly aware of and interested in the affective consequences of attachments: "Many of the most intense emotions arise during the formation, the maintenance, the disruption, and the renewal of attachment relationships" (Bowlby, 1977, p. 130). But, as he notes when he continues, " . . . emotions are usually a *reflection* of the state of a person's affectional bonds" (p. 130; emphasis added). For Bowlby, then, affect is primarily a consequence of and clue to the style of attachment. We believe this misses the point that affective responses also play a significant role in *determining* the style of attachment.

The forming and sustaining of meaningful attachments has a good deal to do with affective authenticity in the sense of an openness to one's own feelings and a readiness to respond to another person's feelings. When we speak of patterns of insecure attachment—or defensive processes—we are referring essentially to inauthentic styles of relating. If one holds to the idea that the formation of intimate bonds between two individuals is made possible through affective freedom, in the sense of expressing feelings openly and honestly, affective restriction is a significant form of defense because it creates relational distance. This is seen most clearly in the case of the compulsive self-sufficient/dismissing patterns. The detachment from, and loss of recognition of, one's true feelings results in the inability to endure intimate relationships.

Affective *restriction* is thus the hallmark of insecure attachment. Interpersonally, it becomes an obstacle to genuine relatedness for two reasons. First, insecurely attached individuals express their feelings in very narrowed ways in their relations to the attachment figure. For example, in the case of the anxious/preoccupied patterns, the exaggerated expression of angry yearning and fearsome expectations about being left alone permit only a shallow concern with the other person's feelings. Second, their expression of affect is likely to be so unmodulated that the other person's feelings or point of view is totally lost or at the least not shared.

These general formulations may be instructive as to the nature of patterns of insecure attachment, but they lack the specificity of particular types of defenses, whether the types are defined by a psychoanalytic or an attachment model. But we propose that this lack of specificity is not a deficiency to be redressed by further research and theory, but rather an intrinsic quality of attachment patterns—and of other psychological structures. Isolation of a particular defensive process is misleading and of limited clinical relevance. The implication is that if the defensive process were to be corrected, then the problem will be fixed, the dysfunction cured. For example, Bowlby's theory implies that to correct compulsive self-sufficiency, one must overcome the defensive process of perceptual exclusion of information. Teach the individual to accurately perceive attachment-relevant information and compulsive self-sufficiency will, by definition, disappear. The simplicity of this approach, while appealing, is manifestly too neat to correspond to clinical reality. It cannot correspond to clinical reality because human cognitions, affects, and behaviors do not comprise discrete and autonomous entities.

S E V E N

THE MEASUREMENT
OF ADULT ATTACHMENT

When we began our investigations of the attachment
system in adulthood, our first goal was to design an instrument to capture the varying expressions of attachment in reciprocal relationships between adults. Despite the theoretical and clinical relevance of the
concept of attachment, the systematic study of attachment in
adults had been hampered by a lack of self-report and interview
measures for its assessment. Most existing measures describing
adult relationships lacked the important orientation of security
through a permanent relationship with a particular, responsive
other.

One early clinical test was developed by Hansburg (1972),
who used pictures depicting different separation situations to ap-
praise responses to separation. Its use, however, is restricted to
school-age children and young adolescents. Hirschfeld et al.
(1977) devised a measure of interpersonal dependency containing items that assess attachment. This scale, however, confounds
the concepts of attachment and dependency, a distinction made
by Ainsworth (1972) and Gewirtz (1972).

Two attachment interviews deserve special attention. Henderson, Duncan-Jones, and Byrne (1980) constructed an interview schedule to evaluate the availability and perceived adequacy
of an individual's attachment relationships. As we discuss in detail in Chapter 10, Henderson's approach assumes that an individual's attachment relationships can be defined as a subset of
his or her social support or affiliative network. Similarly, Heard

and Lake (1986) proposed that attachments be understood as "preferred relationships" within a social network. The underlying assumption of these approaches is that attachment relationships serve the same functions and exhibit the same characteristics as affiliative relationships. The distinguishing characteristic of attachment would, therefore, be the degree to which the relationship fulfilled affiliative needs: Within these approaches "attachment" becomes simply a name for the closest affiliative relationship.

This assumption of an intensity continuum between affiliation and attachment is lent credence by the fact that in our culture the two types of relationships are generally achieved through the same mechanism, that is, the development of close personal relationships. Additionally, relationships cannot be uniquely compartmentalized according to function; rather, one relationship may serve multiple functions. For example, a "best friend" may meet intimacy needs by functioning as a confidante, affiliative needs by functioning as a companion in social activities, and support needs by functioning as a resource in times of crisis. This example also illustrates the inadequacy of a unidimensional, intensity continuum for characterizing and differentiating relationships: The function(s) of the relationship must also be taken into account.

Within studies of infant–parent attachment, the attachment system has a unique function and specific identifying criteria. As we discussed in Chapter 1, we restrict the use of the term "attachment" to dyadic relationships in which proximity to a special other is sought and maintained to provide a sense of security. The principal function of adult attachment is protection from danger. One of the principal differences between adult and infant attachment is that adults recognize more subtle dangers to existence than infants, specifically, threats to the individual's self-concept and integrity (Hinde, 1975; West, Livesley, Reiffer, & Sheldon, 1986). The principal differences between attachment and affiliative relationships are *functional,* with affiliative relationships serving to meet intimacy needs and to promote exploration and expansion of interests from the secure base provided by attachment.

Therefore, we define attachment relationships for the purpose of investigation primarily in terms of function (achievement of felt security) rather than in terms of structure (specific behaviors or form of relationship). Any relationship may have an attachment component to the degree that the relationship promotes security. A relationship becomes an attachment relationship when the primary purpose of the relationship is the provision of security. In related research (see Chapter 10), we have demonstrated that adults differentiate close relationships based on the expectation of finding security within the primary attachment relationship. In contrast, expectations for shared intimacy and confiding were common to both the primary attachment relationship and to close friendships. To minimize confusion between attachment and affiliative components, we have focused our investigations of adult attachment on the primary attachment relationship.

The second interview we want to note particularly is the Adult Attachment Interview (AAI; George et al., 1985). Theoretically, our work is in close accordance with the AAI. The AAI yields three primary classifications of an adult's "present state of mind in regards to attachment": dismissing, autonomous, and enmeshed. Each subject is also classified for the presence or absence of features of unresolved/disorganized mourning associated with loss or trauma in early attachment relationships. The primary differences between our measurement instruments and the AAI are technical rather than theoretical. The obvious difference is the structure of the investigation; the AAI is a semistructured interview, while we use a self-report questionnaire. The focus of questioning is also different. The AAI investigates the pattern of past attachment relationships to parents to draw inferences regarding the person's working model of attachment. Additionally, the patterns of attachment derived from the AAI are validated against the patterns of infant attachment derived from Mary Ainsworth's Strange Situation Protocol (Ainsworth et al., 1978). Thus, although the goal of the AAI is to define the adult's "present state of mind in regards to attachment" (Main et al., 1985, p. 68), the empirical validation relates to parental rather than reciprocal attachment. Our instruments investigate the characteristics and quality of behaviors relating to current, reciprocal attachment to another adult.

In addition to these two interviews, there are now several

other instruments, using various measurement strategies, that are based explicitly on attachment theory. Most of these instruments focus on the assessment of the patterns or styles of attachment (Hazan & Shaver, 1990; Sperling, Sharp, & Fishler, 1991; Bartholomew, 1990). It is not our purpose here to provide a thorough review of existing methodologies, but rather to describe our own work in this area. These different approaches should not be viewed as competing, but rather as complementary, offering the opportunity for studies of convergent validity.

GUIDING PRINCIPLES

We wanted an instrument, firmly grounded in attachment theory, to capture the expression of attachment criteria in adulthood. We were immediately faced with a foundational question: Did we want to attempt a dimensional assessment of the characteristics that define attachment relationships, or did we want a categorical assessment of varying styles or patterns of adult attachment? We decided, perhaps not surprisingly, that what we wanted was to avoid putting all our measurement eggs in one basket. Therefore, we developed scales both to assess the definitional characteristics of attachment and to assess attachment patterns. Our initial efforts focused on adults who were currently in a relationship that could be described as an attachment relationship. We later dealt with the problem of characterizing the attachment characteristics of those adults who are without an attachment relationship.

Following the strategies of Loevinger (1957) and Jackson (1971), our empirical method included attention to substantive validity, rational and empirical strategies to assure structural validity, and the achievement of an internally valid and reliable instrument before proceeding to test external validity. This approach emphasizes the importance of psychological theory in generating an item pool; suppression of response style variance; substantive generalizability and scale homogeneity; and the importance of fostering convergent and discriminant validity at the beginning of test development. This construct-oriented approach is preferable to more empirically based strategies, which often neglect the theoretical foundation for the constructs being measured. Our first task was the operational definition of each construct to be measured.

THE DEFINING CHARACTERISTICS OF ADULT ATTACHMENT

We defined adult attachment operationally in terms of the *criteria* that differentiate adult attachment from other social behaviors and the *provisions* supplied by attachment relationships. Weiss's (1982) application of attachment theory to adults struck us as a particularly cogent approach to defining criteria. The work of Henderson (1977) provides the most useful description of what attachment relationships give to people.

Weiss, on the basis of his work with primary group relationships, concluded that adult attachment bonds largely fulfill the following criteria for attachment (1982, p. 173):

1. In the face of stress, individuals will attempt to seek contact with their attachment figures.
2. Increased comfort and diminished anxiety occur in the presence of the attachment figure.
3. Separation or threat of separation from the attachment figure causes "discomfort and anxiety on discovering the attachment figure to be inexplicably inaccessible."

We developed separate scales for each of these three criteria of attachment, and following Rutter (1981), named them proximity-seeking, secure base effect, and separation protest, respectively.

Secure base effect is a central feature distinguishing attachment from other affectional relationships. *Proximity-seeking* and *separation protest* are behavioral manifestations of these features. The secure base effect in infants is very dependent on the physical proximity of the attachment figure: As Ainsworth's studies demonstrated, infants will display uncertainty and restrict their exploratory behaviors when the mother leaves the room. In adults, security is still a feature of the attachment system, but is more dependent on the internalized representation of the attachment figure. Thus, exploratory behaviors and adaptive responses are more independent of the attachment figure's presence.

In the adult, as in the infant, stressful experiences will activate the attachment system. Stressful experiences are perceived as threatening, that is, as diminishing security. In response to stressful situations, one may try to avoid separation from the attachment figure (i.e., *separation protest*) or, if not with the attachment figure, one may seek his or her presence (i.e., *proximity-seeking*). Again, the securely attached adult relies on the internalized representation of the attachment figure as well as his or her physical proximity, so there will be less urgency to the need and less tendency for separation protest and proximity-seeking to overwhelm other coping responses.

In speaking about attachment, Bowlby (1973) has characterized the relationship as one that is persistent over time and differing situations. There is the expectation, in other words, that the relationship to the attachment figure will be relatively long-lived or permanent. We included a fourth scale, *feared loss of the attachment figure,* to tap the ability to sustain confidence in the permanence of the attachment relationship.

Anticipated permanence of the relationship (the converse of feared loss) is characteristic of adult attachment because adults are not time-bounded, but rather orient themselves to past, present, and future. Security, therefore, can only be found in a relationship that ensures future as well as present security. The securely attached adult will believe in the permanence of the relationship and not be preoccupied with fears of loss of the attachment figure or of harm befalling the attachment figure, and consequently the self.

Bowlby (1969/1982) and Hinde (1982) noted that the principal function of adult attachment is to provide protection from danger through the maintenance of a mutually reinforcing relationship with a particular other adult. For adults, the expectation is that an individual will both require an attachment figure (i.e., a provider of security) and be able to function as an attachment figure. In adults, attachment is usually reciprocated. We included *reciprocity* as a fifth criterion to distinguish adult attachment from other forms of attachment (e.g., parental) that are complementary.

Adult attachment relationships can therefore be distinguished from general social relationships using five criteria: proximity-seeking, secure base effect, separation protest, anticipated permanence of the relationship, and reciprocity. To complete the definition, the role of attachment for the individual, that is, the unique provisions offered by attachment, also must be specified.

In general, attachment provides a unique relationship with another individual who is perceived as available and responsive and who is turned to for emotional and instrumental support. Bowlby (1973) points out that not only must the attachment figure be available but that he or she also needs to be perceived as willing to act responsively. To recognize this potential asymmetry, we developed separate scales for the *availability* and the *perceived responsiveness* of the attachment figure.

Finally, it was necessary to take into account the work of Henderson (1977) and Henderson, Duncan-Jones, and Byrne (1980) demonstrating the independence of availability and perceived adequacy of attachment. An individual might have a high level of accessibility to the attachment figure but perceive this level as inadequate. This suggests that making use of an attachment relationship may be a function of the individual's personality characteristics. Certain attributes are likely either to hinder the individual's use of available attachment relationships or make for ineffective use of these relationships at times of stress. We decided, therefore, to include *use of the attachment figure* as a separate scale.

We began scale development with these eight characteristics to describe the hallmarks of a relationship with the primary function of providing security through a stable dyad, that is, of a reciprocal attachment relationship between adults.

THE PATTERNS OF ADULT ATTACHMENT

As we detailed in Chapter 5, Bowlby (1977) describes three patterns of insecure attachment: anxious attachment, compulsive self-reliance, and compulsive care giving. As well, Bowlby (1973) has referred to a balance between anxious and angry attachment from which an ambivalent pattern arises. We briefly review here the primary features of each pattern.

Compulsive Self-Reliance

Those whom Bowlby (1977) and Parkes (1973) have described as compulsively self-reliant give self-sufficiency a central place in conducting their lives. Bowlby (1977, p. 207) stated, "So far from seeking the love and care of others, a person who exhibits this pattern insists on keeping a stiff upper lip and doing everything for himself whatever the conditions." The defensive flavor of this apparent "switching off" of attachment feelings is obvious. Closeness to others is shunned lest the underlying attachment needs are awakened and place the person in a position of too great vulnerability.

Compulsive Care Giving

In the compulsive care-giving pattern, close relationships are established but always with the person in the giving role, never allowing himself of herself to receive care. As Bowlby (1977) points out, the typical childhood experience of these individuals is to have been prematurely forced into caring for a parent and/or sibling. Thus, the personal history has not only reconciled this person to the imperative of attachment feelings, albeit not their own, but more significantly to losing their self for another. In this respect, the pattern reminds one of Winnicott's (1965) "false self."

Compulsive Care Seeking

Compulsive care seeking has much in common with what Bowlby called "anxious attachment." According to Bowlby (1977, p. 207), this pattern derives from experiences leading an individual to doubt the attachment figure's availability and responsiveness, and so "to live in constant anxiety lest he lose his attachment figure and, as a result, to have a low threshold for manifesting attachment behavior." As a consequence of this anxiety, these individuals attempt to confirm their security with the attachment figure in a concrete manner by displaying urgent and frequent care-seeking behaviors.

Angry Withdrawal

Perceived inaccessibility of the attachment figure gives rise not only to anxiety but also to anger. Analogous to Ainsworth and Bell's (1970) Group C children, who seek contact with mother but are also contact-resisting and angry during the reunion episode procedure, adults can direct both anxious and angry behaviors toward their attachment figures. Like Fairbairn (1954), Bowlby interprets the main source of anger directed toward an attachment figure as a reaction to frustration of attachment desires. Even when the individual attempts withdrawal rather than taking the anger out directly, there is usually, if not always, an important admixture of anger—it is angry or spiteful withdrawal.

To capture these patterns in a questionnaire, we began by identifying the component facets of each pattern. We identified three facets of *Compulsive Self-Reliance:*

1. Avoids turning to the attachment figure for help.
2. Avoids giving the attachment figure affection or closeness.
3. Uncomfortable with attachment figure needing him or her.

Similarly, we identified three facets of *Compulsive Care Giving:*

1. Always places highest priority on needs of other.
2. Has feelings of self-sacrifice and martyrdom.
3. Provides care whether or not it is requested.

The three facets of *Compulsive Care Seeking* are:

1. Defines life in terms of problems requiring assistance to solve.
2. Defines attachment relationship in terms of receiving care.
3. Expects attachment figure to assume responsibility for major areas of life.

Finally, the three facets of *Angry Withdrawal* are:

1. Negative reactions to perceived unavailability of attachment figure.

2. Negative reactions to perceived lack of responsiveness of attachment figure.
3. Generalized anger toward attachment figure.

These facets were used as the basis of item generation.

EMPIRICAL VALIDATION OF THE QUESTIONNAIRE

We have conducted a number of studies to test the validity and reliability of the instrument we call the Reciprocal Attachment Questionnaire (RAQ). The RAQ includes scales assessing the characteristics of adult attachment and scales assessing the patterns of adult attachment. We began with approximately 300 items. The items were derived primarily from clinical experience and secondarily from relevant clinical literature. Items were edited using a number of criteria such as content saturation, judged freedom from response bias, and unitary structure. Through painstaking—and painful—empirical studies we have narrowed this questionnaire down to 43 items tapping five dimensional scales of three items each, and four pattern scales of seven items each.

Because our studies focus on reciprocal attachment only, subjects were given specific instructions for identifying their attachment figure. The attachment figure was defined as someone with whom they plan to continue sharing their lives; someone to whom they were very close and with whom they could share their problems and most private feelings; and someone upon whom they could depend for comfort and turn to to be held at times.

We recognized that an individual might have more than one relationship with attachment components, but it was also assumed that there would be a hierarchy among these relationships. Therefore, the individual was asked to select the one person to whom he or she felt especially close. We defined an attachment figure as a peer (not a member of the family of origin), with whom there is usually a sexual relationship, and with whom a relationship has been sustained for at least 6 months.

We began our empirical work with a study conducted using a sample of 78 university student volunteers enrolled in an undergraduate psychology course (West & Sheldon, 1988). We used this sample to determine an early version of the four pattern scales, containing ten items each. In this study, we were primarily concerned with the internal coherency or reliability of each scale and the discriminant characteristics of the scales.

We then used these 40 questions for the pattern scales with a much larger set of questions for the dimensional scales in later studies. The first questionnaire for these studies contained 139 attachment-related items, with each item associated with only one scale. A 5-point response scale was used, ranging from "strongly disagree" to "strongly agree." All original item sets included both positive and negative statements of the construct. This questionnaire provided the foundation for studies with three sets of subjects, including both psychiatric patients and nonpatients, to confirm the structural relationships, to further refine the scales, and to investigate test–retest reliability.

The first set of subjects consisted of 101 nonpatients recruited from the volunteer service department of a large teaching hospital. The second set consisted of 68 outpatients from the psychotherapy program in the same hospital. All patients had non psychotic diagnoses including personality disorders and anxiety disorders. Patients gave written consent to participate, following an explanation of the purpose and protocol of the study. In order to have a uniform population for each scale, all subjects with any missing data were eliminated from the analyses. The final number of subjects in these two sets were 89 nonpatients and 63 patients.

Based on results from these two sets of participants, the questionnaire items were edited and revised to improve psychometric properties (e.g., scaler internal reliability, interscale correlations, and interitem correlations) while maintaining theoretical consistency. The revised set of items was then used for a mail-out survey within the Calgary community. Survey distribution was roughly stratified by selecting four communities based on community profiles prepared by the City of Calgary. The communities included an upper-middle-class neighborhood near the university, two middle-class neighborhoods in different areas of Calgary, and a working-class inner-city neighborhood. Although we did attempt a stratified distribution, the resultant study population is not a probability sample, and therefore no inferences can be drawn from the pattern of responses obtained in this study to patterns that would be observed in any wider population (i.e., mean scores cannot be interpreted as *norms*). The purpose of these studies was to test *questionnaire* characteristics, not to obtain normative values.

In addition to the attachment items and the demographic items, the community survey also included the Symtom Checklist-90 — Revised (SCL-90-R; Derogatis, 1977) to provide a general screen for probable psychopathology. One hundred forty-nine responses were received, a response rate of 10%. Thirteen subjects were eliminated from the analyses: 12 because their scores on the Global Symptom Inventory (GSI) of the SCL-90-R were greater than 1.5 standard deviations above the mean for our respondents, and 1 who was under age 18. We felt that high scores on the GSI, indicating an elevated probability of current psychopathology, would confound results within this survey group. Subjects eliminated by reason of GSI score did not exhibit any significant demographic differences from remaining subjects, by t-test with $p \leq 0.05$. Thirty-five of the 136 subjects agreed to participation in a retest survey and completed the attachment questions again approximately 4 months following the initial survey.

We have reported on each of these studies in detail in the professional literature; we refer the interested reader to those articles for details of the methods and results (West, Sheldon, & Reiffer, 1987; West & Sheldon, 1988; West & Sheldon-Keller, 1992). In general, for each study, we investigated the means and standard deviations for individual items and scales, to ensure that none of our scales are susceptible to bias from floor or ceiling effects and that there is adequate item variability. We eliminated items with high correlations with other items, so that the items designated for each scale exhibit general congruency without redundancy. We assessed the internal reliability and test–retest reliability of each scale. We also assessed the correlations between the scales and the underlying construct validity (using factor analysis) of the instrument.

These statistical investigations revealed a number of practical problems with our original instrument. These problems are related to the format of investigation. A self-report questionnaire is susceptible to some well-known biases and limitations, such as the possibility of answers biased by social desirability, the difficulty of probing related concepts without undue repetition, and the necessity to deal in generalities that will be applicable to a broad range of people but that cannot describe the unique characteristics of individual situations.

We had to deal with a number of these issues in determining the final content of the RAQ. First, the measurement of *reciprocity* seemed unduly influenced by social desirability: The majority of respondents in both the patient and nonpatient samples had scores indicating a high degree of reciprocity in the relationship. This was true even for those subjects with scores indicating high *compulsive self-reliance*. Based on evidence from several studies, we decided that we could not assess reciprocity validly and reliably in this format. We therefore eliminated reciprocity from our dimensional scales.

A second problem was the degree of correlation between some of the dimensional scales. *Secure base* and *separation protest* consistently exhibited a high correlation ($> .70$), as did *responsiveness* and *availability*. Despite the theoretical distinction between these concepts, we found that empirical separation in a self-report questionnaire was not possible.

In studies of infant attachment (Ainsworth & Bell, 1970), secure base is demonstrated by behavior in the presence of the attachment figure when there is no threat or "strangeness." In such situations, the presence of the attachment figure promotes exploration. Separation protest, in contrast, describes the infant's behaviors when the attachment figure leaves the physical proximity of the infant. In this situation exploration does not occur and the infant protests physical separation from the attachment figure.

Attachment relationships in adults are based largely on internal working models of an attachment figure. The quality of the internalized model will be only partially reflected in behaviors, for behaviors are multidetermined. In a similar vein, Bretherton (1985, p. 12) has observed that the decrease in overt attachment behaviors in older children "does not, however, imply the waning of the attachment system."

In adults, the demonstration of secure base and separation protest depends largely on an investigation of the individual's internal constructs about the degree to which the attachment relationship promotes exploration and the importance ascribed to physical proximity to the attachment figure. Behavioral items, which are the most appropriate items for a questionnaire format, can tap these constructs only indirectly and awkwardly. We hypothesize that the high correlation between secure base and separation protest in our studies is due primarily to limitations of the measurement technique rather than to convergence of the underlying constructs. The separate assessment of *secure base* did not add sufficient unique information to the assessment of *separation protest* to justify its retention as a separate scale. We therefore eliminated *secure base* as a scale.

The case is somewhat different theoretically for *availability* and *responsiveness*. In speaking about availability, Bowlby (1973, p. 202) stated that "the word 'available' is to be understood as implying that an attachment figure is both accessible and *responsive*" (emphasis added). The high interscale correlation in our studies supports Bowlby's formulation rather than our own. We therefore combined these scales, giving greater weight to the responsiveness items and designating the new scale *available responsiveness*.

Factor analytic studies confirmed the theoretical structure of the RAQ. For the five dimensional scales, a four-factor solution, with orthogonal rotation, was optimal. All factors had Eigenvalues greater than 1, indicating that both factors contributed significant independent information to the overall instrument. The six items comprising the scales of *use of the attachment figure* and *available responsiveness* are the only items with coefficients greater than .47 on the first factor. The three items with significant loadings on the second factor comprise the scale of *feared loss*. All of these items had coefficients of at least .72. Items loading on the third factor with coefficients of at least .75 are all from the *separation protest* scale. The fifth factor contains items from the scale of *proximity-seeking*, each with a coefficient of at least .57.

We also performed a factor analysis with the five scale scores. In this case, a two-factor orthogonal solution was optimal; again each factor had an Eigenvalue greater than 1. The scales of *use of the attachment figure* and *available responsiveness* comprised the first factor, each with coefficients greater than .80. The scales of *proximity-seeking* and *separation protest* comprised the second factor, with coefficients greater than .76. The scale of *feared loss* had a coefficient of .56 associated with the first factor and one of .61 associated with the second factor. Feared loss thus seems to be a pivotal concept, empirically as well as theoretically.

Factor analysis of the pattern scales yielded two significant factors. The first factor contained the patterns associated with avoidant attachment: *compulsive self-reliance* and *angry withdrawal*. The second factor contained the patterns theoretically associated with anxious attachment: *compulsive care seeking* and *compulsive care giving*.

The primary reliability and validity statistics for the dimensional scales of the RAQ are contained in Table 7.1; the statistics for the pattern scales can be found in Table 7.2. These statistics are based on a sample that included 136 nonpatients and 110 psychiatric patients.

Using box plots to graphically represent the median and the 95% confidence interval of the median for each scale, we examined the ability of the scales to discriminate between patients and nonpatients in our sample. *Compulsive Care Giving* was the only scale that did not significantly differentiate patients from nonpatients. This finding suggests the importance of attachment in understanding certain types of psychiatric illness, but more definitive work is needed to clarify this important issue. We know, for example, that our patient and nonpatient groups differed in age. We also observed some interaction between scores on the attachment scales and gender. Finally, we do not have definitive diagnoses for the patients in the sample, nor can we state definitely that none of the nonpatients had an undiagnosed psychiatric illness. We know that the patient sample did not include any patients with psychotic disorders and that most of the patients had received clinical diagnoses of mood disorder, personality disorder, and/or adjustment disorder. We also know that the nonpatients retained in the sample had acceptable scores on the GSI of the SCL-90-R. While these observations give us some confidence

TABLE 7.1. Reliability and Validity Statistics for the Dimensional Scales of the Reciprocal Attachment Questionnaire

	Reliability		Factor analysis		Scale correlations			
	Internal	Test-retest	Factor 1	Factor 2	Available responsiveness	Feared loss	Proximity seeking	Separation protest
Use of the attachment figure	.74	.77	.53	−.73	.55	.32	−.18	.18
Available responsiveness	.85	.68	.81	−.32	1.0	.57	.16	.40
Feared loss	.83	.81	.83	.04		1.0	.34	.52
Proximity seeking	.71	.82	.48	.75			1.0	.45
Separation protest	.78	.76	.75	.34				1.0

TABLE 7.2. Reliability and Validity Statistics for the Pattern Scales of the Reciprocal Attachment Questionnaire

	Reliability		Factor analysis		Scale correlations		
	Internal	Test-retest	Factor 1	Factor 2	Angry withdrawal	Compulsive care giving	Compulsive care seeking
Compulsive self-reliance	.73	−.77	.90	−.19	.61	−.24	.08
Angry withdrawal	.80	−.54	.87	.27	1.0	.08	.36
Compulsive care giving	.70	−.79	−.21	.85		1.0	.37
Compulsive care seeking	.77	−.75	.32	.78			1.0

in the results to date, we plan further studies to define more precisely the discriminant ability of these scales.

The questions associated with each scale in the final version of the RAQ are given in Appendix A. The RAQ should be useful as a tool to enrich understanding of attachment relationships. At this time, there are no normative scores for these scales. Clinicians and researchers can use the scales to profile individual patients and to assist in comparative studies of clinical groups. As we discuss in Chapter 8, the specification of attachment dysfunctions may be particularly pertinent to the understanding of personality disorders.

DEVELOPMENT OF A QUESTIONNAIRE FOR THOSE WITHOUT AN ATTACHMENT RELATIONSHIP

When we began development of the RAQ, we also began development of a questionnaire appropriate for adults who lacked an attachment relationship. Our focus for this questionnaire is those adults who consistently lack an attachment relationship, rather than those who have recently (i.e., within the last year) suffered the loss of an attachment figure. In all our studies, we included directions for determining the person most likely to be classified as an attachment figure. For those people unable to identify such a person in their lives, the instructions were to proceed to a separate section of the questionnaire. That section contained the items for the scales we had identified as central to an assessment of avoidant attachment.

To develop scales to assess avoidant attachment, we turned not only to attachment theory, but also to the field of personality theory, in particular to the characterization of the schizoid personality. Since 1925, when Kretschmer (1925) made his interpretation of schizoid personality, object relations writers have conceived of the schizoid individual's relational dilemma as synonymous with the oscillation of an "intense longing for love" with "detachment from the outer world (Guntrip, 1969, p. 44). As this statement suggests, it is the tension between opposing tendencies that lies at the heart of schizoid pathology. Even those who are at the extremity of withdrawal and detachment have a deep desire for closeness. This characterization of the schizoid individual's relational dilemma is reminiscent of Bowlby's distinction between the compulsive self-reliant individual's public self-sufficiency and an underlying longing for attachment. To capture this oscillation, we developed separate scales for each component and named them *maintains distance in relationships, places a high priority on self-sufficiency,* and *desires close affectional bonds.*

Two other significant features mark avoidant attachment. For attachment theorists, object relations theorists, and personality theorists alike, fear of rejection is an important dynamic underlying an individual's withdrawal from close relationships. We therefore designated a fourth scale, *fear of hurt or rejection,* to tap this feature.

Finally, Main et al. (1985) have argued that the avoidant response is adaptive in the sense of offering the best possibility of achieving proximity to a caregiver who rejects a "demanding" child but is willing to maintain proximity as long as the child is undemanding. For such a child, the expression of attachment behaviors becomes not a means of obtaining security, but rather a threat to security. For such individuals who have become adults, the idea of being close to someone is likely to arouse intense fear. So we developed a fifth scale, *attachment relationship is a threat to security,* to assess the extent of this fear.

Despite the fact that the study of avoidant attachment was proceeding at the same time as the study of reciprocal attachment, we are not as far along in the empirical testing of these scales. There is a very simple reason for this: Avoidant attachment, as we have defined it, is relatively rare. Most adults can identify someone who is appropriately called an attachment figure. Therefore, only a small minority of subjects in each of our studies completed the avoidant attachment questionnaire.

To date, we have a composite sample of 63 subjects who have completed the avoidant attachment questionnaire. Of these, 31 are psychiatric patients and 32 are nonpatients. The mean age of these respondents is 33.2 years ($\pm$ 2.43 years); 22 are male and 41 are female.

Following the same strategy as we detailed above for the reciprocal attachment scales, we have confirmed the internal reliability and construct validity of four of these scales. One scale, *fear of hurt or rejection,* exhibited such substantial overlap with the other scales that we eliminated it as a separate scale.

These scales exhibit satisfactory empirical characteristics. Alpha coefficients of reliability range from .72 to .89, indicating a high level of structural coherence for each scale. Item–scale correlations show that each item is empirically as well as conceptually related to the other items of the scale for which it was developed. The results of the factor analysis reflect the contrasting components of a wish for an attachment relationship versus fear of and withdrawal from such a relationship. Factor 1 has high positive coefficients for the scales of *maintains distance in relationships* and *attachment relationship is a threat to security,* while Factor 2 has a high positive coefficient for *desire for affectional bonds* and a negative coefficient for *high priority on self-sufficiency.* The reliability and validity statistics for these scales are summarized in Table 7.3. Appendix B gives the items comprising each scale.

Using the subjects who were psychiatric patients, we tested the ability of these scales to discriminate those patients with a diagnosis of schizoid and avoidant personality disorders from other patients. One scale, *desire for affectional bonds,* did not differentiate the two groups: All patients scored relatively high on this scale. But the other three scales did differentiate the schizoid and avoidant disorder group from the group with other disorders. These results indicate that schizoid and avoidant patients may be best characterized as both desiring an attachment relationship and fearing intimate ties. It is the tension between these opposing tendencies that lies at the heart of avoidance of intimacy.

FUTURE DIRECTIONS

Inevitably, we chaffed against the restrictions inherent in self-report questionnaires, including the inability to include any open-ended probes; the conflict between behavioral items with high reliability, and attitudinal and emotional items with high theoretical validity; the problem of socially desirable responses; and the inability to further explore contradictory responses.

TABLE 7.3. Reliability and Validity Statistics for the Scales of the Avoidant Attachment Questionnaire

| | Internal reliability | Factor analysis | | Scale correlations | | |
		Factor 1	Factor 2	Distance[b]	Desire[c]	Threat[d]
Self-sufficiency[a]	.74	.35	−.69	.18	−.26	.28
Distance[b]	.88	.86	.22	1.0	.20	.46
Desire[c]	.72	.22	.85		1.0	−.11
Threat[d]	.79	.78	−.29			1.0

[a]Places priority on self-sufficiency.   [c]Desires close affectional bonds.
[b]Maintains distance in relationships.   [d]Attachment threatens security.

We turned naturally to the development of a semistructured interview to address these problems. Soon after we began work on the interview, one of us was trained by Dr. Mary Main in the rating of the AAI. From the AAI, we adapted several theoretical concepts and measurement strategies, particularly relating to the use of *coherency of discourse* as a marker of security of attachment.

Our Reciprocal Attachment Interview, though more satisfactory than the questionnaire, was lengthy to administer and score. We still sought a more efficient method for discriminating different styles of reciprocal attachment. In particular we were interested in developing a technique based on projective techniques with content and style analysis by multiple raters.

Once again, our work was assisted by the work of others in the field: in this case, the earlier work of Hansburg (1972), who used attachment-relevant pictures as the basis for a series of questions probing the separation anxiety of children and adolescents. The latest tool in our battery of methods to investigate adult reciprocal attachment uses attachment-relevant pictures to elicit stories from our subjects. Combining approaches used in the attachment-centered work of Hansburg and Main, and the "classical" strategies of the Thematic Apperception Test (TAT, Shneidman, 1951) and Rorschach (Klopfer, Kelley, & Davidson, 1942), we focus on both the *content* and the *style* of the responses. Our hypothesis is that subjects react to, interpret, and explain the pictures according to their personal internalized working model of attachment.

Currently, we present each subject with three pictures relating to childhood (see Appendix C). The subject is asked to construct a story about each picture; the interviewer sometimes supplies nondirectional prompts to encourage elaboration. The responses are tape-recorded and transcribed. The typed transcripts are then independently reviewed and rated by three raters—a technique that will be immediately familiar to those who have been trained to rate the AAI.

To give a flavor of the variation we see, we can contrast the stories constructed by two subjects in response to the child-in-bed picture. Each subject is a young man, in his mid-20s, living in a metropolitan area, and is a college graduate with a "middle-class" life-style. Subject A constructed this story to describe the picture:

"Well this is . . . um . . . I'd say it was bedtime, going to bed, going down for the count at night and you just want one final hug from Mom and you're doing anything to stop having Mom leave and turn the lights out and you have to go to sleep. The stories are over and she's read you the chapter, or whatever book she was reading to you, or what not, and you just get that final hug in before you get to sleep for the night."

Compare Subject A's story to the one constructed by Subject B:

"Well, the child is obviously, seems to be looking for a hug probably at bedtime. The mother doesn't seem to be really making any move towards the child . . . (*long pause*). . . . The drawing is interesting, there's no faces but the child still seems to appear sad, . . . um yah . . . the mother could be punishing him . . . uh . . . holding back affection. Probably not, it's probably more that she doesn't respond quickly or well to affection."

These responses illustrate the *qualitative* differences in stories. These differences are evident even to an untrained, or un-attachment-oriented, ear. Our goal is to construct ratings that will quantitatively reflect these qualitative differences.

Our rating criteria continue to evolve as our experience broadens, but we have not changed or significantly modified our original orientation. We use five primary categories for rating the pictures. For the two pictures depicting a child and an adult interacting, we first rate simply on *Presence of Attachment Content*. By that we mean, briefly, "Is there any content in the response that relates to *security* invested in the relationship?"

The next rating category is *Responsiveness of the Caregiver,* that is, "What does the content of the story reveal about how the adult responded to the child?" We have observed four distinct variations in this category: appropriate responsiveness is directly cited; no responsiveness is mentioned; the adult is characterized as unresponsive; the adult is overtly characterized as punitive.

The third rating category is *Internalized Secure Base* and is rated only for the picture without an adult figure. This again is a content focused rating and asks the question, "How are the child's feelings and thoughts construed?"

The fourth rating shifts the focus from the content of the response to the semantic style of the response. Like Mary Main's *Coherency* rating, ours is based on Grice's (1975) four maxims of coherent discourse. We use the five markers of incoherency developed by Main and her colleagues for the AAI: unlicensed violations of Grice's maxims of quality, quantity, relation, and manner; and instances of dysfluency and distancing. These five ratings are intermediary steps only, to sharpen and clarify the rater's final assessment of the coherency of the response.

The fifth and final rating again evokes an AAI rating: *Lack of Resolution of Mourning.* The criteria for this rating are not easily summarized. The best broad statement we can make is that this rating addresses the question of the degree to which the subject gives evidence of attachment responses being heavily influenced by past loss or losses. A positive rating for *Lack of Resolution of Mourning* is suggested, for example, whenever the coherency of response to the picture depicting the ambulance scene is notably less than the coherency of responses to the other two pictures.

Finally, each rater uses these ratings to estimate the predominate reciprocal attachment pattern of the subject. To date, this estimate is done entirely heuristically—we do not have an algorithm for translating ratings into attachment patterns.

Clearly, our work with this assessment technique is in its infancy. We have not yet conducted any studies of reliability or validity. Rather, we are still refining our assessment technique. The refinement of our methods and the development of our theory has become an interactive process: We remain firmly grounded in object relations theory and the attachment system, but we increase both our understanding and the sensitivity of our scoring as we work with these instruments.

Using this technique in conjunction with our questionnaire and the work of other investigators, we are slowly evolving a picture of how an adult's internalized working model of attachment is expressed within his or her current primary reciprocal relationship.

EIGHT

PERSONALITY
DISORDERS RESEARCH

Since 1980, when the American Psychiatric Association (APA) published the third edition of its *Diagnostic and Statistical Manual of Mental Disorders* (DSM-III), and 1987, when the APA published its revised third edition (DSM-III-R), there has been an outpouring of research on the validity and reliability of diagnosis for personality disorders, including a new professional journal, the *Journal of Personality Disorders*. Earlier editions of the DSM, particularly in its aspects pertaining to "character disorders" made free—and to many critics, freewheeling—use of psychodynamic constructs. Faced with the practical problem of providing "clear descriptions of diagnostic criteria in order to enable clinicians and investigators to diagnose, communicate about, study, and treat the various mental disorders" (American Psychiatric Association, 1987, p. vii), the authors of DSM-III undertook to define personality disorders strictly in accordance with the principle of phenomenological description. This approach is theoretically neutral: All that need be assumed is that personality disorders are aggregates of certain regularities of functioning expressed in consistent behaviors. Clinicians and investigators of quite different theoretical orientations can agree on the description of such regularities as long as they are not required to commit themselves to any theoretical position concerning the processes that give rise to them.

What is wrong with this picture? Perhaps nothing is essentially wrong. Ainsworth's methodology for classifying attachment patterns is a rather good example of a phenomenologically based classification method. Patterns of attachment are defined by aggregates of observable behaviors found to be stable across subjects and studies. Why such patterns should exist is, in some sense, a separate question. Nonetheless, Ainsworth's empirical method for classifying attachment behaviors, although not dependent on a theoretical structure for measurement, was guided by an underlying theory of attachment that lent coherency to the general approach.

In contrast, DSM-III-R's methodology for classifying personality disorders disclaims any such underlying theoretical orientation. But several characteristics of the schema suggest that an underlying theoretical structure does exist. First, DSM-III-R organizes personality disorders into three clusters and, further, labels these clusters. This organization betrays an underlying theory about differential commonalities among the disorders. The label of Cluster 1 implies that, as a group, these disorders are differentiated from other disorders by odd or eccentric behaviors. Cluster 2 disorders are differentiated by dramatic, emotional, or erratic behaviors. Cluster 3 disorders are differentiated as "individuals who appear to be predominantly anxious or fearful" (Webb, DiClemete, Johnstone, Sanders, & Perley, 1981, p. 128). These labels illustrate one danger in not making the theoretical stance explicit: which two labels (Clusters 1 and 2) refer to behaviors, it is not clear whether the third label (Cluster 3) refers to behaviors or to affects. Thus an individual who is fearful or anxious could seek to accommodate this fearfulness in odd or eccentric ways—leading to a confusion between placement in Cluster 1 and placement in Cluster 3.

Second, criteria are not necessarily exclusive to one diagnosis. Not only do common criteria again betray underlying assumptions about the convergence of disorders, but they cross the boundaries of clusters, indicating that more than one pattern of association among disorders underlies the classification scheme.

The third piece of evidence is based on the observation that antisocial personality disorder is both the most reliable to diagnose and shares common features with all other Cluster 2 disorders. The important point to note here is that these common features do *not* constitute part of the operational definition of antisocial personality disorder. The operational definition (i.e., the criteria) focus on the features *unique* to antisocial personality disorder. The diagnosis of antisocial personality disorder thus comes closest to making the underlying theory explicit. The inclusion of criteria specific to antisocial personality disorder and the exclusion of criteria shared with other Cluster 2 disorders implies a hierarchical or decision-tree structure. The first level of differentiation is the cluster level; within the cluster, specific disorders are further differentiated by how the cluster characteristics are expressed in different behavioral patterns.

Thus, DSM-III-R's paradigm of organization is primarily hierarchical categorization with differentiation beginning at the cluster level and proceeding to the diagnosis level. The weaknesses of the organizational paradigm used in DSM-III-R can be summarized briefly as follows:

1. At the initial level of differentiation among clusters, the definitions are not mutually exclusive.
2. For most diagnoses, the specific criteria are composed of a combination of cluster criteria and disorder criteria. Antisocial personality disorder is the notable exception.
3. More than one theory of association seems to be operating, as evidenced by the sharing of common criteria by diagnoses in different clusters.
4. The implicit hierarchical structure from cluster to individual diagnoses is neither clearly formulated nor justified.

AN ALTERNATIVE PARADIGM

Hierarchical structures are important and common structures in organizing information. Notably, the prototype of scientific classification systems, the taxonomy of the animal world, is hierarchical, proceeding from *kingdom* through *phylum, class, order, family, genus* to *species*. But the use of hierarchical classifications is by no means universal. Many taxonomies are based on a *dimensional* classification system. So, for example, in anthropology, cultures are not compared in regard to placement in a hierarchy but in terms of similarities or differences in a number of specific areas, such as familial structure, means of obtaining food, religious systems, and so on. Although there may be correlation between various dimensions of interest, cultures that are similar on one dimension will not necessarily be similar on other dimensions. The crossing of criteria between clusters in DSM-III-R suggests that a dimensional organization is more appropriate than a hierarchical classification for personality disorders. In a similar vein, Millon (1987, p. 110) has proposed that "it would make good scientific and practical sense if certain specific realms were consistently addressed, for example, affective response, style of cognitive functioning, pattern of interpersonal behaviors, self concept, and so on." These "specific realms" can be understood as dimensions for classification.

Dimensional systems have traditionally been favored by psychologists (Widiger & Frances, 1985; Endler & Edwards, 1988). These systems vary greatly in the number of dimensions specified, the structured correlation among the dimensions, the labeling of the dimensions, and their correspondence to traditional diagnostic structure (Frances & Widiger, 1989). Nonetheless, the limitations of categorical models has made dimensional systems increasingly attractive. As Frances and Widiger (1989, p. 252) note, "It is likely that a dimensional approach will eventually become a standard method for personality diagnosis because the personality disorders do not have the internal homogeneity and clear boundaries most suited for classification in a categorical system."

Additionally, to speak of personality disorders at all is to speak in terms of difficult interpersonal relationships. There is substantial agreement that the interpersonal dimension, traditionally identified as an affiliation dimension, is of particular relevance to DSM-III-R, Axis II disorders. Widiger and Frances (1985) give a strong statement of this position:

> An interpersonal nosology is particularly relevant to personality disorders. Each personality disorder has a characteristic and dysfunctional interpersonal style that is often the central feature of the disorder. There is also some empirical support for the hypothesis that a personality disorder is essentially a disorder of interpersonal relatedness. (p. 620)

Several ways in which the interpersonal domain is explicitly relevant to personality disorders can be specified. We are particularly interested in four of the disorders: schizoid, avoidant, dependent, and borderline. These four disorders, which cut across the three clusters in Axis II, are among the most prevalent, among the most difficult to treat (particularly borderline) and have been extensively studied and written about in the professional literature.

In regards to these disorders, in particular, and the entire spectrum of Axis II disorders, in general, the interpersonal domain is relevant to:

1. Existing criteria: Seven of the eleven personality disorder diagnoses contain criteria that explicitly refer to these types of relationships. Only histrionic, narcissistic, compulsive, and passive aggressive do not contain criteria referring explicitly to disturbed interpersonal relationships. Additionally, only low self-esteem for avoidant and lacks self-confidence for dependent are defined without reference to interpersonal relationships.

2. Presenting complaints: Impoverished or disturbed interpersonal relationships are frequently the presenting complaint of patients subsequently diagnosed as personality-disordered; therefore these relationships are of particular value in organizing initial knowledge about an individual.

3. Etiology: The important role that emotionally significant bonds play in the development of personality and the maintenance of psychological well-being has been acknowledged across many fields, including psychoanalytic theory and developmental psychology.

Although difficult interpersonal relationships have gained wide acceptance as the hallmark of most personality disorders, DSM-III-R's formulations of the types and functions of interpersonal relationships are generally vague and imprecise. The nature of these difficulties with relationships are specified in broad terms only, for example, "one or two close friends" in the instance of schizoid personality disorder. DSM-III-R refers to a specific type of relationship for only one personality disorder, antisocial, noting that the individual has "never sustained a totally monogamous relationship" (American Psychiatric Association, 1987, p. 346). In general, though, the characterizations are not distinct or precise enough to be clinically useful.

In these circumstances, we have proposed that dysfunctions of the attachment system can be used to achieve greater specificity of symptomatology in this area (West & Sheldon, 1988). By definition, attachment relationships are important and enduring features of an individual's pattern of interpersonal behaviors. Thus, a consistent framework for identifying patterns of insecure attachment should contribute substantially to understanding the personality-disordered individual's difficulties with forming and sustaining interpersonal relationships.

Indeed, studies of an association between attachment problems and personality disorders have recently been appearing in the literature. Examples include several studies by Livesley (and his colleagues) on traits typical of personality disorders. In one study (Livesley, 1987) descriptors culled from the psychiatric literature were grouped into 79 categories which were then placed into 1 of 12 personality disorders by clinicians. In a list of six typical characteristics of schizoid personality disorder, avoidant attachment ranked second. In another study of personality pathology in a general population sample of 3,256 subjects, Livesley, Jackson, and Schroeder (1989) identified 15 factors, accounting for 75% of the total variance, to organize 100 scales of personality traits and behaviors. One of the factors, Insecure Attachment, subsumed the traits and behaviors of *separation protest, secure base, feared loss, proximity-seeking, intolerance of aloneness,* and *need for affection.*

In a related study of dimensions associated with dependent personality disorder (Livesley, Schroeder, & Jackson, 1990), these investigators report that two orthogonal factors were identified in studies with a general population sample and a clinical sample. In each study, these factors accounted for approximately 71% of the variance and exhibited congruent loadings of trait and behavioral scales. Factor 1, labeled Insecure Attachment, subsumed the scales of *separation protest, secure base, proximity seeking, feared loss,* and *need for affection.* This factor accounted for 39% of the variance in both studies. The four scales comprising the second factor, labeled Dependency, were *low self-esteem, sub-missive, need for advice and reassurance,* and *need for approval.* This factor accounted for 33% of the variance in the general population study and 32% of the variance in the patient study. In an earlier study by Hirschfeld et al., (1977), similar factors were identified: Factor 1, labeled Emotional Reliance on Another Person, contains items relating to feared loss of loved ones, fear of abandonment, need for close relationships, feelings of help-lessness when alone, and general support seeking. Factor 2, la-beled Lack of Social Self-Confidence, contains items relating to advice seeking, submissiveness, and lack of confidence in one's own decisions. Factors 1 and 2 resemble the Insecure Attachment and Dependency factors found by Livesley et al. (1990).

Among other efforts in this direction is an article by Pilko-nis and Frank (1988), who conceptualize their finding of avoidant and dependent personalities among unipolar depressed patients in terms of Bowlby's opposing attachment patterns of compul-sive self-reliance and anxious attachment, and an article by Melges and Swartz (1989), who characterize the borderline individual's intense, unstable relationships in terms of oscillations of attach-ment. Further, Livesley and Schroeder (1991) reported the results of a study on traits typical of Cluster B personality disorders. A panel of psychiatrists considered attachment problems — in par-ticular, the tendency of borderline patients to regress when sepa-rated from their attachment figures — to be a highly prototypical feature of the disorder.

Thus, in the recent literature concerned with personality dis-orders, the clinical value of attachment theory to the understand-ing of personality disorders has attained some prominence. One need not seek further than avoidant personality disorder for the implications of insecure attachment for personality disorders.

AVOIDANT PERSONALITY DISORDER

One of the most notable differences between the DSM-III and the DSM-III-R in Axis II criteria is the elimination of the moti-vation for emotional involvement (desire for affection and ac-ceptance) from the description of avoidant personality disorder.

Instead, DSM-III-R places much of the emphasis upon the Avoidant personality-disordered individual's lack of comfort in social situations and his or her lack of skill as a group member. The desire for, yet fear of, dyadic intimacy is replaced by this lack of comfort in unfamiliar social relationships. It might appear arbitrary to differentiate between nondyadic sociability and dyadic intimacy, but we suggest that these are two different kinds of developmental achievements.

By not making this distinction in its description of avoidant personality disorder, the DSM-III-R appears to exclude individuals who have social skills but little or no confidence that they will find security with a significant other. This point is clear if one accepts the probability that there is no necessary connection between comfortable sociability and the capacity to form and sustain close attachment relationships. For example, in clinical practice we commonly hear patients say that they have many friends but no one with whom they feel a special closeness. What is characteristic of an attachment relationship, and obviously impossible to obtain in general social relations, is the feeling of security arising from proximity to a particular and preferred other. The inability to rely upon another person for security may, therefore, have clinical significance for avoidant personality disorder which is very different from that of discomfort in general social relationships.

We investigated the idea that desire for, but fear of, attachment relationships is a more cogent criterion than social discomfort and timidity for avoidant personality disorder in a study of patients attending the outpatient psychotherapy unit of a large teaching hospital (Sheldon & West, 1990). In this study, 47 (24 males and 23 females) patients who had received a clinical diagnosis of avoidant personality disorder completed a brief questionnaire that rated desire for an attachment relationship, fear of an attachment relationship, and level of social skills. No one in this group of patients was living in a marital type relationship; all responded negatively to the question, "Is there someone in your life now that you would describe as your attachment figure?" None of the patients had experienced recent (less than 1 year) loss of an attachment figure, indicating that the lack of an attachment figure was not situationally determined, but rather reflected a long-standing pattern.

The results supported our hypothesis that desire for, but fear of, an attachment relationship is more clinically relevant to avoidant personality disorder than lack of social skills and comfort. Attachment desire for these individuals necessarily implies no expectation of fulfillment and a lack of confidence in the attachment figure's permanence and responsiveness (feared loss of the attachment relationship). This conflict is resolved behaviorally by an avoidant reaction.

The inability to feel secure within an attachment relationship is present to some degree in other personality disorders, although the way in which it is articulated and expressed varies from one disorder to another. Over the last 5 years we have used the attachment instruments described in Chapter 7 to study the empirical association between various personality disorders and the components and patterns of attachment. To demonstrate the significance and potential of this approach, we include here two studies: the first highlighting the comparative strength of association between borderline personality disorder and attachment characteristics, and the second highlighting the discriminant power of attachment concepts in relation to avoidant, schizoid, and dependent personality disorders.

BORDERLINE PERSONALITY DISORDER

Three of the positive DSM-III-R diagnostic criteria for borderlin personality disorder (BPD)—a pattern of unstable and intense relationships, difficulty tolerating being alone, and frantic efforts to avoid real or imagined abandonment—are defined with reference to interpersonal behavior. Indeed, evidence has gradually accumulated to an impressive degree that interpersonal dysfunctioning is a predominant feature of borderline individuals. Surveyors of research on borderline personality disorder, such as Dahl (1990), Westen (1990), and Links (1990), conclude that unstable and intense relationships is one of the most sensitive borderline criterion. From an attachment standpoint, the interpersonal difficulties of borderline individuals may be seen as intimately bound up with this dilemma: chronic failure to experience felt security in the face of the inability to be alone. Their lack of belief in the reliability of an attachment relationship leads to an anxious enmeshment with their attachment figure as well as to doubts about the desirability of the relationship.

We conducted a study to assess the discriminatory ability of attachment, compared to other functional and social characteristics, in relation to the diagnosis of borderline personality disorder. As described in detail elsewhere (West, Keller, Links, & Patrick, 1993), a sample of 146 patients was drawn from a year's total consecutive admissions to treatment in the outpatient psychiatric clinic of a large teaching hospital. The total number of outpatients admitted for treatment within the time frame of this study was approximately 200. This sample therefore represented a consecutive survey of 73% of patients admitted for outpatient psychiatric treatment during the time of the study.

Out of a total sample of 146 patients, 115 had current attachment figures, according to their own self-reports, based on criteria supplied by the investigators; that is, a marital or intimate relationship, usually but not necessarily sexual, of at least 6 months duration with an adult who was not a member of the family of origin or a child of the participant. These 115 participants constituted the sample for this study and were administered the following questionnaire battery: the Millon Clinical Multiaxial Inventory (MCMI; Millon, 1983) for diagnosing personality disorders; the Symptom Checklist (SCL-90-R; Derogatis, 1977) as a measure of pathological syndromes; and three measures of the interpersonal domain, the Reciprocal Attachment Questionnaire (RAQ), Mehrabian's Affiliative Questionnaire (MAQ; Mehrabian & Karonzby, 1974), and the Interpersonal Dependency Questionnaire (IDQ; Hirschfield et al., 1977).

Of the 115 participants with a current attachment figure, 74% (n = 85) were female and 26% (n = 30) were male. A total of 47 females (55% of the females) and 5 males (17% of the males) scored above 74 on the MCMI borderline scale. Because of this bias, and because of the low number of male subjects with borderline diagnosis, we discuss the results for females only. The participants remaining in the sample were therefore 85 females psychiatric outpatients with a current identified attachment figure; 38 of these subjects (45%) scored less than 75 on the MCMI borderline scale (BR); 16 subjects (19%) scored between 75 and 84 on the borderline scale; and 31 subjects (31%) scored above 84 on the borderline scale.

The results indicated that neither the measures of more general interpersonal characteristics (MAQ, IDQ) nor the measure of psychopathology (SCL-90-R) demonstrated any statistically significant association with borderline personality disorder. Only three scales from the RAQ—feared loss of the attachment figure, compulsive care-seeking, and angry withdrawal—were significantly related to borderline personality disorder. All three scales exhibited linear trends: the group scoring above 84 on the borderline scale had the highest means; the group scoring 75 to 84 had the intermediate means; and the group scoring below 75 (no borderline diagnosis) had the lowest means. No other scale on any of the instruments had a p value less than .01.

To investigate the relative importance of these three scales to the determination of borderline personality diagnosis by the MCMI, a multivariate analysis of variance was performed. One significant canonical variable was identified. The correlations of the three dependent variables with the canonical variable were: feared loss $= -0.86$; compulsive care seeking $= -0.67$; angry withdrawal $= -0.64$. feared loss, therefore, has the predominant role in interpretation of the canonical variable, with the other two scales having approximately equal effects. This suggests that the attachment feature most characteristic of borderline disorder is feared loss of the attachment figure and the attachment relationship.

The analyses presented above provide a statistically precise demonstration that, of the scales measuring psychopathology and interpersonal characteristics, only three scales—each related specifically to adult attachment—are significantly related to a diagnosis of borderline personality disorder in female patients. The high feared loss is characteristic of anxious attachment as identified and defined by Bowlby (1977). This characteristic forms the underlying strata or raison d'être of borderline personality disorder. The two attachment behavioral patterns significantly related to the disorder reveal the contradictory and ill-fated defenses with which the individual attempts to bind and limit the anxiety. The conjunction of *compulsive care seeking* and *angry withdrawal* echoes the vacillation between extremes that is clinically characteristic of this disorder and is captured in the DSM-III-R diagnostic criteria. It is worth noting here that, despite the diagnostic overlap inherent in the MCMI (because one item can load on more than one scale), no other personality disorder sub-sample in our complete subject group exhibited this conjunction of compulsive care seeking and angry withdrawal.

In the case of female borderline patients, "angry yearning," to use Bowlby's (1963) term, appears to be the central affect around which their relationships are organized. The yearning component leads to an enmeshed relationship with the attachment figure; female borderline individuals attempt to confirm their security with their attachment figure in a concrete manner by displaying urgent and frequent care-seeking behaviors. The search for security, however, is repeatedly frustrated and gives rise to angry withdrawal. Their hypersensitivity to threats to the continuity of the attachment relationship is of special importance. It is tied up with anticipatory anxieties over being able to meet their needs for security, as well as with the noted oscillations of urgent care seeking and angry withdrawal.

AVOIDANT, SCHIZOID, AND DEPENDENT DISORDERS

To investigate the usefulness of attachment characteristics in sorting out issues of diagnostic overlap among these disorders, we turned to our full sample of 115 patients.

Demographically, three-quarters of our sample were females; about half of our sample were between the ages of 35 and 50; most had at least a high school education; and approximately half were currently living in a marital-type relationship.

The MCMI has been cited as corresponding particularly well to DSM-III-R diagnoses of schizoid, avoidant, and dependent disorders (Widiger & Frances, 1987). Based on the MCMI scores, we established four diagnostic groups:

1. No schizoid, avoidant, or dependent disorder: $N = 53$
2. Schizoid and/or avoidant disorder but not dependent: $N = 18$

3. Dependent disorder only: $N = 18$
4. Schizoid and/or avoidant with dependent disorder: $N = 26$.

We were not able to separate schizoid and avoidant disorders as there was almost complete diagnostic overlap between these two disorders. As Figure 8.1 reveals, males and females did have different patterns of disorder in this sample. Females are over-represented in the categories that include a diagnosis of dependent disorder and underrepresented in the schizoid and/or avoidant diagnostic category. Because of this, we included gender as a factor in all analyses. No other demographic factor showed a strong relationship to diagnostic category.

The general technique of multivariate analysis of variance is wellsuited to address the questions of interest for this study. The specific structure of the analysis was chosen to reflect the underlying theoretical relationships of the attachment scales. The dimensions of attachment constitute a substrata underlying the patterns of attachment, which represent specific dysfunctional forms of relating to an attachment figure. The dimensions of attachment are therefore logically prior to the patterns of attachment. The patterns of attachment, on the other hand, are "more

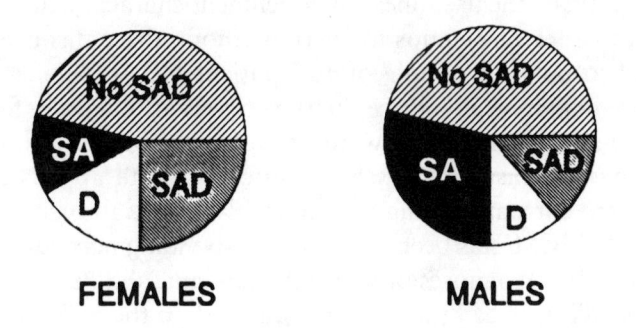

FEMALES   **MALES**

FIGURE 8.1. Distribution of diagnostic categories, by sex. No SAD = no scores above 84. SA = scores above 84 on schizoid and/or avoidant but not dependent. D = scores above 84 on dependent but not schizoid or avoidant. SAD = scores above 84 on schizoid and/or avoidant, *and* dependent.

visible," as organized behaviors, and more congruent to usual diagnostic criteria of symptoms and syndromes.

The results are summarized in diagrammatic form in Figure 8.2. Of the demographic variables, only gender demonstrated a strong association with the variables of interest. The best interpretation of the interaction between gender and diagnostic category is that *females* who were in the *dependent disorder group* tended to have higher scores on *compulsive care giving* than the other subjects, while *males* who were in the *dependent disorder group* tended to have lower scores on *compulsive care giving* than the other subjects. This result must be accepted with extreme caution for males, as there were only 3 males in the study in the Dependent Disorder Group. A high score on the dimensional scale measuring *proximity seeking* was associated with high scores on the pattern scale measuring *compulsive care seeking,* which in turn was associated with the personality disorder category of mixed *schizoid, avoidant, and dependent disorders.*

Low scores on the dimensional scale measuring *use of the attachment figure* was associated both with high scores on the pattern scale measuring *compulsive self-reliance* and with the personality disorder category of *schizoid and/or avoidant disorder. Use of the attachment figure* was the dimensional scale most strongly related to *compulsive self-reliance,* and therefore had the strongest effect on the association between *compulsive self-reliance* and the *schizoid–avoidant* category.

Low scores on the dimensional scale of *availability* were strongly associated with high scores on the pattern scale of *angry withdrawal*. These scales seemed to have the least association with the diagnostic categories.

The results of this study reveal clear patterns of association among the variables. These associations lend support to the theoretical proposition that attachment problems underpin several existing personality disorder diagnoses, and that these diagnoses can be more precisely and coherently defined by explicit reference to attachment dimensions and patterns as diagnostic criteria.

From these results it appears that the minority of patients with "clean" diagnoses of schizoid or avoidant personality disorders correspond very well to the attachment pattern of compulsive self-reliance. But something much more complicated is

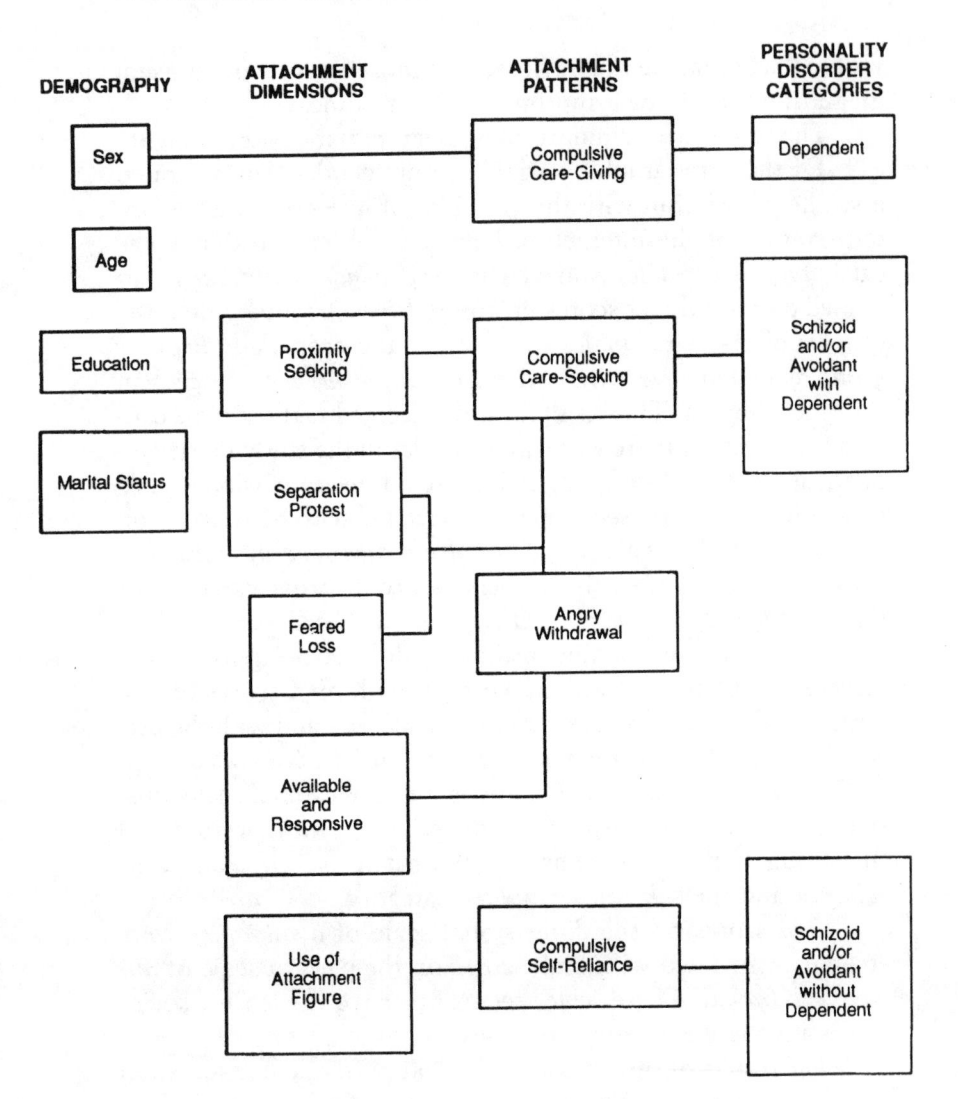

FIGURE 8.2. Diagrammatic summary of the associations among four classes of variables: demographic, attachment dimensions, attachment patterns, and categories of personality disorder.

going on with the diagnosis of dependent disorder. Despite the prima facie linguistic correspondence between dependency and compulsive care seeking, there is no clean empirical correspondence. Instead, females in the Dependent Disorder Group exhibited a pattern of compulsive care giving. This finding is worth highlighting as it emphasizes the point made by feminist psychological writers that "dependency" in women is more closely associated with construing one's life as *taking care of others* rather than construing one's life as *needing to be taken care of* (Stiver, 1990; Eichenbaum & Orbach; 1985).

CONCLUSION

In the decade since DSM-III was published, the accomplishments of personality disorder research in establishing these disorders as distinct categories are not impressive (Livesley & Jackson, 1992; Perry, 1992). If these disorders overlap as much as the research appears to indicate, we need to face the question of whether they can be separated into 11 discrete categories at all. In this regard, the working group on personality disorders often seem to mistake the capacity to advance what a categorical system of personality disorders ought to be for the capacity to produce empirical support for such a system. And when it comes to the practical problem of treating personality-disordered individuals, the current diagnostic system is of questionable usefulness in helping clinicians to target treatment processes and goals.

The observation of Widiger (1992) that the field of personality disorders requires clarification of the major dimensions bearing on it are applicable. A dimensional approach holds promise for a genuine articulation of the problem of overlap among personality disorders. The observed overlap is not primarily a consequence of measurement problems (i.e., issues of reliability), but rather an inevitable consequence of constructs underlying the measurements. To increase reliability by eliminating overlap is to sacrifice validity for reliability. The alternative approach is to increase validity and reliability by clarifying the underlying constructs and establishing operational definitions (cf.

criteria, phenomenological descriptions) that directly address these constructs. The results of our research described above and that of others (e.g., Livesley, Jackson, & Schroeder, 1991) indicate that the attachment construct contains information that is essential to understanding and classifying personality disorders.

NINE

ATTACHMENT
AND PSYCHOTHERAPY[1]

Of the many aspects of attachment theory, Bowlby paid the least attention to a theory of psychotherapy. He made only one reference to the therapeutic implications of attachment theory in the second part of *The Making and Breaking of Affectional Bonds* (1977) which he later elaborated upon in *A Secure Base* (1988b). But if Bowlby himself did not leave us a complete theory of an attachment-based psychotherapy, he did provide the core concept around which such a theory could be organized. In *Pathological Mourning and Childhood Mourning* (1963), Bowlby demonstrated convincingly that yearning for an experience (a close loving relationship with a parental figure) that never happened or that happened only inconsistently is the basic problem in neurotic difficulties and personality disorders. In addition, Bowlby did elaborate in a most lucid manner the consequences of the individual's failure to master this "lost" relationship in terms of patterns of insecure attachment. Taken together, these two ideas are highly relevant to the description of an attachment theory of psychotherapy.

THE THERAPIST AS A PROTECTIVE FIGURE

Although, as we saw in Chapter 5, Freud (1926) placed felt loss of the object at the center of his revised theory of anxiety, this accent on object ties was not incorporated into psychoanalytic technique. Rather, psychoanalytic therapy continued to locate the therapeutic process in the individual's intrapsychic machinery. Interpretations of this intrapsychic content that hit the mark (i.e., led to insight) remained the primary determinant of change.

Today one hears less about individuals' intrapsychic conflicts or of their failure to adequately control unacceptable impulses, and hears more about their natural relatedness tendencies and the environmental deficiencies that thwart them. Theorists of the developmental arrest or object relations point of view have indicated that the individual is from the beginning more social and able to initiate social interaction than Freud supposed (Fairbairn, 1952; Winnicott, 1965; Balint, 1968). This view gave much greater attention to the protective function of the therapeutic setting than it previously had received in traditional psychoanalytic theory. What Bowlby (1988b) and Ainsworth (1989) describe as the secure base provided by the childhood caregiver becomes a compelling metaphor for the therapeutic relationship.

Individuals who come for therapy live with a sense of helplessness in the face of the threat of feared loss and insecurity. The first goal of the therapist is to remove the threat, in so far as possible, and create a "background of safety," to use Sandler's (1960) term. As noted by Bowlby (1988b, p. 140), "Unless a therapist can enable his patient to feel some measure of security, therapy cannot even begin." Reliance upon the therapist as a protective figure nullifies the individual's sense of helplessness and establishes "a secure base from which he can explore the various unhappy and painful aspects of his life, past and present, many of which he finds it difficult or perhaps impossible to think about and reconsider without a trusted companion to provide support, encouragement, sympathy, and, on occasion, guidance" (Bowlby 1988b, p. 138). As we discuss later in this chapter, the therapist's creation of a safe environment enables the individual to recapture and cope with disavowed feelings associated with caregiver responsiveness failures.

Bowlby (1988b, p. 140) stresses the role of the therapist as "analogous to that of a mother who provides her child with a secure base from which to explore the world." As Modell (1976) observes, both the "ground rules" of psychotherapy and the therapist's basic stance contribute to the individual perceiving the therapist as an attachment figure, that is, as someone who is stronger and/or wiser. The therapeutic relationship is an unequal one in which individuals reveal everything about themselves while the therapist's communications are not self-revealing. This necessary communication differential establishes the therapist as the helper and the individual as the one to be helped, a "tilted relationship analogous to a parent–child relationship" (Greenacre, 1954, p. 672). The therapist's emotional attitude also fosters an atmosphere akin to that described by Winnicott (1986) as "holding." This attitude includes a genuine interest in the patient, reliable availability, and a wish to help. At the same time, the therapist tolerates the patient's painful affects and tries to remain friendly and nonretaliatory in the face of the full force of these feelings.

The therapeutic relationship encompasses the simultaneous presence and interaction of two forces: the patient forming an attachment to the therapist and the therapist's willingness to be perceived as an attachment figure. It is tempting, of course, to identify the patient's attachment to the therapist with the child's attachment to the parent, even if this connection is only intended analogously. The temptation appears to be irresistible when instead of attachment the term "dependency" is used to describe the nature of the therapeutic relationship. Dependency inevitably makes one think of regression; the therapist–patient relationship is thus conceived as bringing modes of relatedness into play that otherwise manifest themselves in the parent–child relationship. Some eminent analysts—among them Balint (1968) and Winnicott (1965)—have expressed or hinted at their belief that the role of the therapist is literally akin to that of a maternal caregiver. Mitchell (1988, p. 170) suggests that this view leads the object relations theorist into regarding the patient "as fixed in developmental time and awaiting interpersonal conditions which will make further development possible. . . . What was missed is still missing and needs to be provided in the form in which it was missed the first time around." In this view, then, the therapist functions as a reparative parental figure, providing relational experiences that were absent during the individual's childhood.

The individual as infant is a metaphorical offspring of the object relations view in which, as we have just seen, the therapist is portrayed as a reparative parental figure. Here the desire for attachment is depicted in terms of regressive infantile long- ings or as a symbolization of the earliest mother–child relation- ship. Mitchell (1988, p. 156), in commenting on this tendency to collapse adult attachment desires into infantile fixations, ob- served: "Relational needs which might reasonably be regarded as aspects of all adult relationships, the longing to be held and cherished, are depicted as regressive symbiotic yearnings, un- resolved residues from earliest childhood." Or in Bowlby's (1977, p. 203) oft-quoted words, "Whilst especially evident during ear- ly childhood, attachment behavior is held to characterize human beings from the cradle to the grave. . . . There is nothing intrin- sically childish or pathological about it."

If the essence of the object relations point of view is that the therapist restores missing parental provisions, the essence of the attachment view is that the therapist offers a different way of relating to the individual. Not only is the individual seen as requiring something new from the therapist—the therapist be- ing a "good" attachment figure—but this kind of need is not in- terpreted as regressive. The acceptance and affirmation of the individual's desire to form an attachment to the therapist, then, is an important (or even the foremost) concern of therapists whose work is influenced by Bowlby's developmental perspective.

This line of thought is fully congruent with Malan's (1979) precept that only negative transference reactions require interpre- tation, thus leaving the positive transference reaction as an unin- terpreted and essentially ambiguous backdrop in therapy. For many individuals who have denied the significance of their at- tachment desires and who have also evaded their import in rela- tion to the therapist, it is unlikely to be helpful to have these desires interpreted as nothing but vestiges of infantile needs. Such a reductionistic stance on the part of the therapist would leave renunciation of these so-called infantile desires as the only path open to the individual.

The position we favor is to understand that what the in- dividual experiences as an intense longing for closeness is reflecting one polar element of an inner attachment drama. Within this in- ternal drama, we can recognize the concurrence of two aspects of a conflictual situation: desire and fear. The desire component, as mentioned above, is essentially a longing for meaningful relatedness. The fear component of the drama arises when expression of the attachment desire is suffused with anxiety about the individual's own vulnerability and anxiety about the reliability of the other person's responsiveness. Our therapeutic approach to this desire–fear attachment drama is to separate the desire from the fear, leaving the desire component as an uninterpreted ground against which the fear component can be examined as figure.

In actual practice, some individuals come into therapy ready to use the secure base provided by the therapist to change their lives. As Bowlby wisely notes (1969/1982, p. 82), life teaches a great deal in that later life may entail "some major change in environment or in the organism: we get married, have a baby, or receive a promotion at work, or less happily, someone close to us departs or dies, a limb is lost or sight fails." It would be a mistake to think that individuals do not profit from these radical changes in attachment relationships or in themselves. As an example of what can be learned from life experiences, Main (1985) reports on parents who were able to take a second look at their own insecure childhood attachment experiences when they became parents and in so doing managed to come to terms with them. As in all relationships with a trusted companion, an individual may be quite ready to use the therapist as a secure base to hasten or intensify the revision of attitudes about attachment in the direction of secure attachment.

The inability to use the therapist as a secure base can be reasonably considered to derive mainly from the individual's inner attachment drama with its conjunction of desire and fear. The therapeutic task is to unmask this drama.

ENACTMENT[2] AND TRANSFERENCE

Ordinarily, when writers speak of the therapeutic process to uncover this inner drama, they are almost always referring to a sequence that moves from insight to positive changes in behavior. Since the early days of psychoanalysis, the analysand has always "gotten better" in the same way. In hysteria, the therapeutic problem was to secure catharsis so that suppressed emotion could be released instead of converted into bodily symptoms. The process was invariant: recovery during hypnosis of a traumatic incident, expression of "strangulated affect," and disappearance of the symptom for good. When free association later replaced hypnosis, the curative pathway was still the same. Therapeutic work on underlying conflicts allowed more material to emerge, which in turn facilitated greater understanding through interpretation. As time went by, the therapeutic process shifted away from interpretation of meaning or motivation (dynamics) to outside realities, from past problems to present and future prospects. Such changes as are achieved in psychotherapy have thus been conceived to move linearly from attributions of meaning to behavior (insight) outward to subsequent changes in behavior. The unfolding of events in therapy has always been conceived to proceed in the same stepwise sequence: Interpretation provides insight, and insight is later translated into positive actions and new ways of conducting one's life.

The delineation of the sequence of events from insight to behavioral change is fully consistent with the ground rule that the individual postpone making any major life decisions while in therapy. In his *New Introductory Lectures on Psychoanalysis* (1933), Freud introduced this rule in order to create the necessary frustration to propel the analytic process (the formation of insight) forward. Over the years, as the nature of the individual seen in psychotherapy changed (fewer presented with neurotic symptoms and more showed character disorders), the length of therapy correspondingly increased. The length of therapy made adherence to this ground rule of not making major decisions during therapy unworkable. It may well be, however, that the injunction was always more honored in the breach them in the observance because it was basically flawed in principle. The right to make decisions and the need to learn how to do so is crucial in every therapy.

Our experience suggests that another sequence of events in therapy is not uncommon. Just as Bowlby (1973) was careful to show that an individual's working model of attachment evolved from the specific and accurate perceptions of past experiences (*from the outside*), so we have to allow that modification of this model may similarly begin with behavioral change. In this therapeutic sequence, the individual, early in therapy, undertakes a new mode of action. These behavioral initiatives take many different forms, such as applying for a promotion at work, enrolling in a university course, asserting oneself a bit more in social gatherings, and so on. The specific initiative is not as important as the place it assumes in the individual's inner attachment drama. The significance of these actions is that they represent an externalization of the individual's inner attachment drama, or at least some element of it. What has been covert is thereby brought out into the open and made available for exploration by both therapist and individual, including the therapist's inevitable enmeshment as a coactor in the individual's inner drama.

Let us turn again to a clinical example to illustrate how a behavioral initiative reflects a core aspect of the individual's attachment drama.

CASE EXAMPLE

At age 28, Helen was referred by her family physician for generalized anxiety. She was tense, restless, and unable to sleep without a sedative. Helen, the second eldest of four children, had grown up in a family that was chaotic as well as impoverished because of her father's severe alcoholism. The father, a World War II veteran, had been so damaged by his wartime experiences that "he looked and acted like a crazy person." A tormented man, he had, Helen said, "a fanatical look in his eyes" that had terrified her. She described him as "terrifically highstrung, opinionated, and noisy."

Speaking of her mother, Helen described her as "uncompromising and unforgiving." Her idea of being close to someone, Helen said, "was to get someone cornered and put them down." She was always tense and brusque and went about "with a chip on her shoulder." Taken together, the personalities of the parents inevitably translated into their being at one time or another the sadistic aggressor or the hapless victim.

Of her parents' marriage, Helen said that there was no love or affection between them: "They fought all the time." She related that she had never eaten a meal at home when "I wasn't afraid that my father was going to tip the table over and start fighting with my mother." Every time her mother had a quarrel with her husband, she threatened to run away or to commit suicide: "It got so I was afraid to go home after school; I was afraid she wouldn't be there, or worse, that I might find her dead."

Early in therapy Helen recalled one of her most frightening childhood experiences. This experience occurred when her father, with a crazed look on his face, had attempted to choke her mother. In retaliation, the mother had attacked the father with a knife, inflicting lacerations. In relating how her parents' violent and irrational actions had terrorized her, Helen said that she "felt like a child lost in the dark, groping blindly with monsters."

Her brother Danny, 6 years younger, also found the battlefield that was their home life unbearable and understood what it was like to be gripped by fear. Because they shared a common plight, Helen and Danny developed a special bond that provided both with a refuge from their parents' "craziness." Helen became like a mother to Danny, spending many hours playing with him and comforting him when he was upset. By the time Helen was 10, she cooked for him, bathed him, and put him to bed at night. After she began working at age 16, she bought Danny presents and gave him spending money.

Helen left home at age 17 to take a job as a waitress. For several years thereafter she created her own battlefield with sex and alcohol as the main weapons of abuse. She became promiscuous, allowing herself to be picked up by men in singles bars; drank to excess; and consorted with a gang that used drugs. Although she was never in love with a man, she twice lived with men who exploited her. These men were neglectful, and when drunk they turned against her and became abusive. In Helen's words, "I didn't know the difference between being cared for and being exploited and hurt."

She emerged from the downward spiral of her life course with a purposeful determination to change things for the better. Helen said she feared that unless she made something of her life she would fade out just as her parents had done. However, the lack of positive identification figures in her past made it difficult for her to pursue this goal. There was certainly an obligatory "paint-by-numbers" flavor to the way in which Helen constructed her new life: She returned to school, took a secretarial job, found new friends, and then moved to a suburban apartment complex. Out of these actions came a "real" life, together with enough anxiety to prompt her to seek psychotherapy.

As Winnicott (1968) points out, there is value in seeing many symptoms as instrumental to self-cure and thus as basically adaptive in the sense of compensating for disturbed childhood environments. For Helen, the caregiving–rescuer role enabled her to compensate for a chronically chaotic family environment. Her parents' conduct appeared to reflect the belief that the only obligatory requirement of parenthood was to bring children into the world and thereafter to merely sustain them physically. Little in their parenting suggested that they were capable of serving as attachment figures—that is, as figures who are stronger and/or wiser and who are better able to cope with life than their children. For Helen and Danny, the only stable element in their chaotic environment was their attachment to each other. Helen's role of caretaker to Danny was thus a way of coping with parents who had lost control of their own lives and were not in charge of their children's lives. This caretaker role can be seen as an example of what Loevinger (1966) termed a passive-into-active coping strategy whereby the individual achieves a sense of mastery by being an active initiator rather than a helpless victim of a dysfunctional attachment environment.

Later in life, such individuals' working model of attachment includes a view of relationships that stresses the importance of providing care and attitudes that serve to control or deny their own attachment needs. To elaborate metaphorically, this view takes up so much space in the individuals's working attachment model that there is little "room" left to perceive relationships from any other perspective. The tendency of these individuals, whom Bowlby (1977) has called compulsive caregivers, to consistently limit the expression of their own attachment desires while always bestowing care upon others calls to mind the mechanism of projective identification. In this process, the other person becomes a vicarious figure onto whom the individual displaces his or her yearning for love and to whom he or she provides the same care he or she would like to receive himself or herself. Although, in Helen's case, the tie to Danny meant her salvation, playing the role of caregiver became the only vehicle through which she was later able to relate to others. What she received, in other words, she received vicariously through taking care of others. Helen herself recognized this style of conducting her life: "I'm so tired of watching others' live and feeling things secondhand."

Helen, as we have seen, undertook a series of behavioral initiatives in an effort to change her life. In terms of the enactment of Helen's inner drama, these actions represented the desire component of her drama, that is, the wish to do something that was of value to her. But one consequence of her moving forward was that this change itself generated severe anxiety. Discovering the source of this anxiety created an agenda for subsequent therapeutic exploration.

During her adolescent and young adult years Helen had lived recklessly, with much drinking and many sexual relationships. As we have seen, she later initiated various actions to improve her life. The outcome of these actions represented "respectability" to Helen, an attainment her previous behavior had made her view as out of reach. But she also felt that she had used up all of her credit in life and therefore did not deserve a happy life. In this regard, Helen dreamed recurrently that she had committed a crime for which she was forced to run a torturing path, like running a gauntlet. Eventually, Helen's anxiety was relieved by structuring her initiatives to change her life in these terms: "You are trying to build a life without craziness." This theme succinctly captured where she had been and where she hoped to go.

The therapist was also involved as a coactor in Helen's drama. In psychotherapy much of the work, often intensely affect-ladened, centers around the effort to understand and work through the effects that the individual's inner attachment drama has on the therapeutic relationship. In Helen's case, she often both exaggerated her past misdeeds and disparaged herself. Her test of the therapist was to discover whether he (West), a respectable, middle-class professional, would accept her. In this regard, Weiss and Sampson's (1986) theory of therapy is perhaps one of the most significant contributions to the concept of transference in recent years. According to their theory, individuals enter therapy with the hope of disconfirming their pathogenic beliefs.

Their disconfirmation is dependent upon the current emotional interactions between the individual and the therapist in the here and now and is in direct proportion to the manner in which the therapist is experienced as a new and different attachment figure. In Piagetian terms, the therapist's offer of a form of engagement that does not correspond to old relational gestalts compels revision of the individual's model; such revision can be seen as a form of "accommodation" in which pathogenic beliefs change in accordance with new experiential information. This is perhaps the best kind of so-called corrective emotional experience.

The individual's experience of a different and broadened way of relating to the therapist leads to a heightened awareness of the discrepancy between this new relational reality and the deficient emotional environment of the past. Paradoxically, this change in the degree and kind of relatedness to the therapist makes mourning necessary. This happens because, prior to the working through of the relationship to the therapist, individuals have been unable, in one sense, and unwilling, in another sense, to conduct their relationships differently. Now, however, the facilitation of mourning can occur from a position of strength by virtue of the fact that the therapist has become someone with whom the individual can reexperience grief and acknowledge loss. The therapist's presence creates an atmosphere of safety to ease the assimilation of disavowed feelings associated with the memory of painful attachment experiences.

THE FACILITATION OF MOURNING

One of the most outstanding characteristics of object relations based psychotherapies is the neglect of the central significance of mourning in therapy. (Indeed, the term "mourning" cannot be found in the indexes of Guntrip, 1969, and Fairbairn, 1952.) Most analysts who view the therapeutic process as providing a restorative experience for the patient do not appear to consider it important for the individual to also mourn never experienced but longed for closeness with childhood attachment figures. This neglect of mourning is perhaps due to the view that missing parental responsiveness is corrected through a reparative experience with the therapist, thereby making the mourning of what was never experienced unnecessary.

As we noted above, Bowlby (1963) proposed that yearnings for an experience that was missing (a longed-for close relationship with the childhood caregiver) are the basic problem in many psychological disorders. It is certainly true that many individuals who come for therapy have not been able to give up the past, and that in their current relationships they are still searching for an experience that never happened. There has been no reconciliation with their past attachment reality; they have been unable to say "good-bye" to lost attachment figures. Although Bowlby has demonstrated in a most lucid manner the clinical implications of pathological adult mourning, he makes no reference to mourning in his later papers on psychotherapy. This omission is surprising, especially in light of the fact that he identifies the contrasting of experiences during childhood and current experiences with the therapist as one of the major tasks of therapy. This comparing of past and present would almost certainly arouse in the individual painful, depressive feelings. Implicitly, such feelings and mourning are inextricably conjoined.

According to Green (1986), the fundamental organizing principle of contemporary analysis is that it strives to complete a delayed mourning process. Green states, "If one had to choose a single characteristic to differentiate between present-day analyses and analyses as one imagines them to have been in the past, it would surely be found among the problems of mourning" (p. 140). Green suggests here that individuals have not only been unable to master their actual losses but also have been unable to master the loss of that which they have deeply desired but never fully experienced. One of the most important goals of an attachment-based psychotherapy is to help the individual master the consequences of caregiver empathic failures, that is, the persistent inability of the caregiver to have appreciated the child's attachment point of view. Chronic experiences of parental unresponsiveness or rebuff summate and become for the individual miniexperiences of loss. They create relational distance and perpetual feelings of not being understood, and hence loneliness. These "losses" must be mourned.

From the point of view of mourning, therapeutic work is

concerned with the undoing of denied losses so that disavowed feelings—principally anger, guilt, and sorrowful yearning—are recognized and then followed into the childhood past. The process of mourning thus provides a direct pathway to past attachment events. This is important in relation to the current debate concerning the actuality, that is, the historical factuality, of these attachment events. Our interest in history as history presumes that past attachment experiences need to be faced realistically and consciously in order to complete a delayed mourning process. A brief presentation of the conflicting views of the historicity of attachment events may add perspective.

Schafer's (1983) and Spence's (1982) writings on the question of reconstruction emphasize that our remembrance of things past is an act of creation. Therapeutic exploration is not so much a matter of reconstruction (the memory of actual past attachment events) as it is an interpretative version of what actually happened in this attachment past. Throughout therapy, different attachment story lines are created; the individual's attachment history is a constantly changing narrative. In Bowlby's (1988b) view, this narrative mode, in which the individual's attachment history is seen as a series of changing story lines over the course of therapy, ignores the fact that every interpretation of the past has more than just a grain of historical truth. The attachment history is grounded in ineffaceable attachment experiences.

Contrary to the idea of "narrative truth," Bowlby (1979) emphasizes the point that there are actual events that give validation to individuals' accounts of their attachment pasts. He lists threats to abandon a child, threats not to love a child, and threats to commit suicide—all used at times by some parents as a means of control. Exploration, then, attempts to recapture these real events and the real influence of attachment figures upon the individual's working model of attachment.

For example, in therapy, the recall of childhood experiences did not come easily for Helen. By employing the metaphor of "a war zone" to speak for her early family experiences, a context was created for uncovering and finding meaning in these experiences. However, in a case of such massive environmental failure, the exclusive use of a metaphor, no matter how revelatory of the individual's past experiences, runs the risk of trivializing them and lessening their full therapeutic impact. Therapeutic exploration must also attempt to realistically define what actually happened in the individual's attachment past in order for these events to be regarded with conviction by both the individual and the therapist. Therefore, although the image of herself as a refugee from a war zone became a touchstone for Helen's traumatic family experiences, the account of her attachment past was also carefully grounded in the actual events of her childhood.

The mourning process thus leads to the recognition of the reality and consequences of the responsiveness failures of early caregivers. In another sense, it simplifies and organizes the relationships between these prior events and present feelings concerning attachment. The mourning reaction, including grief, anger, and yearning, may be illustrated by the case of Helen. As she began to encompass her losses, she often fell into a sad mood. In some sessions she remained silent and simply weeped after she had untangled the impact of the missing tender relationship with her parents. In other sessions Helen railed against her parents' failure to be attachment figures (someone stronger and/or wiser) for her. By making these feelings conscious, a final settlement of the hurt and sense of loss Helen had felt due to her apparent failure to get the tender attentions from her parents was made.

Helen's efforts to find a set of values to guide her life led to an awareness of the discrepancy between her present life and the nihilistic "nothing has any meaning" chaos of her past. Her discovery of meaning also made mourning necessary. The wasted possibilities and the missed opportunities of the past were deeply felt by Helen. Moreover, she grieved for her brother Danny whose hospitalizations for depression Helen interpreted as a failure to discover meaning in his own life. She came to see that, like the deep and protracted loyalty displayed by Anna Freud and Sophie Dann's (1951) children, she too had continued to feel responsible for Danny's well-being. However, she also came to appreciate the truth that she could no longer appropriately be responsible for her brother's psychological state now that he was an adult. This separation from her brother together with the erosion of her self-definition as a caregiving rescuer led to the recognition of the possibility of a new type of relationship based upon full reciprocity rather than unsatisfactory complementarity.

INSIGHT AND OUTLOOK

Because of incomplete mourning, an individual's awareness of loss is submerged; his or her old griefs, yearnings, and anger are denied; beliefs about attachment are grim and pessimistic; and the whole experience of attachment is narrowed. As we have described, psychotherapy revolves around the therapist providing the individual with a secure base and then helping the individual to bring together attachment experiences, memories, and feelings. When the individual recalls past attachment experiences, these experiences are integrated with expectations concerning significant others in the present, particularly the therapist. Once connectedness between these areas is recognized, an enlarged and more open concept of attachment reality results. Ultimately, conviction and insight appear as the individual in effect is able to say "Now I understand and feel that all of this is true."

In therapy, the individual's affectively charged beliefs about attachment are the focus of exploration. This involves taking a "second look" at what past attachment experiences have done to influence present relationships. By uncovering the secrets and landmarks of their past attachment experiences, individuals can begin to integrate past and present, perception and memory, ideas and affects. Insight, then, is based on understanding the subtle but often painfully obvious effects of caregiver responsiveness failures upon current attitudes toward and expectations concerning others.

The discerning reader will have noticed that this account of insight in terms of enhanced integration comes very close to Main et al.'s (1985) definition of secure adult attachment. Main cogently argues that adult security is the capacity to integrate information relevant to attachment and to accommodate new information so that attitudes and expectations are better adapted to current relational realities. Conversely, insecure attachment results from the distorting influence of "rules" that restrict the flow of attachment information; defensive processes are directed against ideas, memories, and affects or the connection between them.

In conclusion, we wish to emphasize our belief that the development of insight is akin to a creative process in that it consists of the putting together of two previously unconnected frames of reference. In Bowlby's (1988b, p. 139) words; "Once he has grasped the nature of his governing images (models) and has traced their origins, he may begin to understand what has led him to see the world and himself as he does." But, as Koestler (1966) points out, this act of discovery operates in a "Janusian" fashion. Any new awareness derives first from the individual escaping from blind representational alleys and disrupting beliefs that distort the affective appraisal of attachment experiences. Only then can new frames of perception be constructed and coded in such a way that the individual may "feel free to imagine alternatives better fitted to his current life" (Bowlby, 1988b, p. 139).

For a further discussion of attachment and psychotherapy, see Appendix D.

TEN

BOUNDARIES
OF ATTACHMENT

A definition of attachment must deal not only with the components of attachment and their organization but with the problem of differentiating attachment from other types of social relationships that have traditionally been seen as closely related to it. Our earlier consideration of the historical background of attachment theory suggests that Bowlby did not so much discover facts in the field of child development as give them a new interpretation (or reinterpretation). In giving the origin of the child's tie to the mother a new theoretical frame, and by inviting others to share his view that the attachment conception was a better formulation of what they were getting at, Bowlby met, to put it mildly, with skepticism from the defenders of psychoanalytic orthodoxy (Freud, 1960; Engel, 1971). Within academic psychology, various critics of attachment theory had their particular axes to grind—the behaviorists predictably viewed attachment as synonymous with attachment behavior, while others argued or implied that attachment was best represented as a trait (Cairns, 1972; Rosenthal, 1973; Masters & Wellman, 1974).

Ainsworth et al. (1978) stated as explicitly as anyone that "attachment" is not the same thing as "attachment behavior." Ainsworth convincingly demonstrated that the distinction between attachment and attachment behavior is the distinction between attachment as an organizational construct and those diverse behaviors that serve the overall system goal of maintaining a desired degree of proximity to the mother figure. This distinction has held sway because simple logic dictates that *if* attachment is defined as a propensity to seek proximity to a differentiated other that, among other things, directs and helps determine various attachment behaviors, *then* it cannot at the same time be attachment behavior.

Among other concepts traditionally related to attachment, dependency seems to have virtually disappeared from the child development literature as an explanation of the nature of the child's tie with the caretaker. Since, however, clinical theory and practice still make use of the concept of dependency, we shall first briefly consider the features that distinguish it from attachment.

Acceptance of the validity of Bowlby's formulations has led to a disconcerting definitional sprawl. The danger, in this instance, is that the attachment construct is stretched to embrace more and more phenomena. Definitional boundaries become blurred and all close relationships are treated as synonymous with attachment relationships. Something of this nature crept into attachment in the areas of romantic love and social support, where an emphasis upon the similarity of mechanisms for maintaining attachment and other interpersonal relationships has been confused with the functional congruence of these relationships. In this chapter, our second intent is to discuss the boundary problems thus posed.

ATTACHMENT AND DEPENDENCY

As we noted in Chapter 1, the traditional psychoanalytic theory of child development built during the first half of this century rested on three principal pillars. These are the doctrines that the infant is in a state of infantile autism; that feeding (orality) precedes personal relatedness, characterized as dependency; and that the tie between infant and mother is a vicissitude of this basic drive. We have already seen that this approach stands in sharp contrast to that of attachment theory in which the caretaker's presence is primary and is not in the service of satisfying some more fundamental need (in Fairbairn's [1952] phrase, "Libido is not pleasure-seeking but object-seeking").

Today, of course, attachment is being studied as functionally independent of dependency. However, in the 1960s and early 1970s, attachment theorists, such as Ainsworth (1968, 1972), had to explicate the conceptual boundary between attachment and dependency. Because dependency continues to have an important place in the thinking of many clinicians, it may be useful to separate these two constructs conceptually, and thereby provide a basis for comparing their clinical implications.

Ainsworth (1972) specified the following areas of demarcation:

1. Specificity: Attachment is dyadic whereas dependence is generalized.
2. Duration: Attachment is enduring while dependency tends to be transient.
3. Level of maturity: Attachment is desirable and positive at all ages, but dependency implies immaturity.
4. Affective implications: Attachment implies strong affect, especially love, whereas the affective component of dependency is usually not addressed. Gewirtz (1972) has further specified that attachment involves a socioemotional bond, whereas dependency involves an instrumentally reliant bond.
5. Proximity-seeking: In attachment, proximity-seeking is specific to the attachment figure, while in dependency it is more generalized.
6. Learning: Attachment requires some discriminative learning while dependence does not.

As we discussed earlier, the concept of dependence is a central aspect of the object relations perspective. Developments since 1940 show a steady movement toward acceptance of the primacy of relatedness. Although the terms used by object relations theorists to stand for experiences central to development are different from those used by attachment theorists, the importance of the quality of the caretaker–child relationship is not a matter of theoretical dispute. There is a great affinity between the two theoretical systems concerning the kind of experiences that are essential for healthy development. For example, Jones wrote in the preface to Fairbairn's *Psychoanalytic Studies of Personality* (1952) that "Dr. Fairbairn starts at the center of personality, the ego, and depicts its strivings and difficulties in its endeavor to reach an object where it might find support." Yet Fairbairn spoke of the outcome of having experienced a secure relationship with the caretaker as *mature dependence* and regarded *infantile dependence* as the basic cause of neurosis. And Guntrip (1969, p. 214), in speaking of ego weakness, indicated that this condition arose from the individual "having had to grow up, not on the basis of feeling safely in touch and secure in a reliable good relationship with the mother, but on the basis of feeling that his inner self is not understood by anyone." These conceptions of development are very close to the heart of attachment theory, although the choice of terms ("mature dependence," "infantile dependence," "ego weakness") are quite different.

On American soil, Parens and Saul (1971) and Saul (1972), writing within a psychoanalytic ego framework, traced the development and manifestation of dependence throughout the life cycle. Similar to members of the British school of object relations thought, Saul (1972, p. 100) holds that "What is fundamental is the personal interrelationship between child and parents. . . . It is this emotional relationship that facilitates or warps the child's personality by shaping patterns of emotional reactions that will be repeated toward others." This statement is fully consonant with Bowlby's position, and Saul in fact marshaled evidence from ethological studies and Bowlby's own writings to support "the central importance of *dependence* . . . for human development and neurosis" (p. 74; emphasis added). In a curious way, Saul, although very much aware of attachment theory and obviously willing to include its contribution in his own scheme, continued to employ the language of dependence to depict development.

One could say that, within limits, these old dependence theories simply reflect a preference for a certain unit of analysis, always a somewhat arbitrary matter, and need not involve theoretical controversy. (To be sure, the matter appears to have been settled in favor of the attachment position on the development

154

of the bond between caretaker and child.) However, to get away from dependency as a force underlying disturbed adult interpersonal relations is another issue. The successful critique of dependency within developmental psychology has not settled the issue of its place as an explanatory concept of adult psychopathology. For example, in clinical psychiatry Hirschfeld, Shea, and Weise (1991, p. 143) depicted dependent personality disorder "as composed of both excessive attachment needs and excessive instrumental dependent needs." To put the emphasis upon "excessive" in describing attachment needs implies that attachment needs are immature or at least maladaptive—a perspective that is inconsistent with our view that attachment is desirable and positive at all ages. As we have demonstrated, the idea that overly strong dependence in adults reflects developmentally arrested needs is common to many object relations theorists.

Consistent with the point of view that the function of attachment behavior across the life span is to achieve or enhance security through relational proximity to a special person, Bowlby opposed the notion that this need reflects infantile dependency desires. For a long time, as Bowlby (1988b, p. 12) observes, "In clinical circles it has often happened that, whenever attachment behavior is manifested during later years, it has not only been regarded as regrettable but also has been dubbed regressive." If we follow Bowlby, then, we must give a preeminent place to a perfectly appropriate search during adulthood to find security in another person. And if this search for security is fraught with intense fear about losing the security invested in the attachment relationship such that the person displays urgent and frequent care-seeking behaviors, it is unhelpful to collapse this experience into overdependency. As Bowlby (1988b, p. 12) points out, "Dependency always carries with it an adverse valuation and tends to be regarded as a characteristic only of the early years and one which soon ought to be grown out of." As his idea of a more suitable term than "dependence" to characterize this condition, he introduced the concept of "anxious attachment." Bowlby used this concept to forestall the tendency to portray adult attachment needs, even when they are imbued with anxiety, as regressive, immature longings.

ATTACHMENT AND ROMANTIC LOVE

The search to find security in an enduring relationship often begins, at least in Western culture, with romantic love. In the prototypical case, two individuals become intensely absorbed in one another and become the focus of each other's lives. Passion and emotional intensity are central to the experience. Although Hazan and Shaver (1987) suggest that such passionate love and lifelong attachment naturally go together, their argument does not persuade us to think that romantic love is necessarily synonymous with attachment. The sense of security in an enduring pair-bond derives primarily from the reciprocal provision of emotional availability to the partner. Initially, in the formation of such an attachment bond, there is a steep increase in this availability component, evidenced by the mutual desire to be almost constantly in each other's company. Over the course of an attachment relationship, emotional availability is maintained in a sort of "steady-state" fashion, reflected in its relatively narrow band of fluctuation. Romantic love, as anyone who has seen too many operas at an impressionable age can attest, also shows this initial steep increase in desire. Unlike attachment, however, romantic love, as a component of an enduring attachment bond, does not maintain itself in a "steady-state" way, but rather ebbs and flows within a much broader range of variation. Put more prosaically, romantic love is like a searing flame of emotion that may either "burn out" or later give rise to a more enduring bond.

As we suggested above, romantic love can be viewed, particularly in the lives of young people in their late teens and early adult years, as a "gateway" or entrance onto the path that will lead to the later formation of a permanent attachment bond. Movement toward adulthood requires young people to relinquish their parents as primary attachment figures and to overcome the feeling that their parents are more capable (stronger and/or wiser) than they are themselves. As adolescents loosen the ties to their families and begin to depersonalize the standards by which they will conduct their lives, they are apt to experience loneliness and even a sense of emptiness (Perlman, 1988). The need to find someone who makes them feel necessary and wanted becomes predominate as a motivation. Put simply, the young person falls in love in a serious way. This intimacy with another "fosters feelings of security just as might a parent; or, to put the matter another way, contributes to the maintenance of an inner state of well-being" (Weiss, 1991, p. 73). Now, the emotional investment in another that meshes the affectional and sexual truly relegates the parents, to use Weiss's term, to the position of "attachment figures in reserve." Even though these early, first loves are liable to break up, they contribute a significant part to developing a permanent attachment in adulthood because something about intimacy and the importance of meaning something to another person has been experienced.

ATTACHMENT AND AFFILIATION

Because attachment and intimacy needs may be satisfied by the same person (e.g., it is a common expectation in our culture that one's spouse will also be one's best friend), a similarity of mechanisms for maintaining both types of relationships appears to have led to a confusion of the functions associated with the two separate relationships. Researchers focusing on the first issue, the range of relationships relevant to support, generally organize relationships into a network that is *unitary* in structure and *diverse* in intensity or saliency only. In other words, the spectrum of interpersonal relationships, in terms of the ability to provide social support, is assumed to be organized from casual acquaintances, through role-related friendships, to intimate friends and family, including unique attachment relationships (e.g., Scott, 1988; Stewart, 1989). Attachment is assumed to arise from the same needs as other close social relationships, to fulfill the same functions, and to be maintained by the same behaviors, cognitions, and affects.

Henderson's (1977) conceptualization is particularly instructive, for he is one of the few investigators to attempt a systematic research study taking into account attachment relationships in adults. Henderson states (in agreement with Caplan, 1974) that " 'psychosocial supplies' . . . [are] . . . the essential commodity that people obtain from their social network" (1977, p. 187). He further proposes that an individual has "affective attachments" toward members of his or her primary group and "it is from them that his psychosocial supplies are said to be derived" (1977, p. 187). As supporting evidence for his thesis concerning the importance of attachment in adults, Henderson cites the study by Brown et al. (1975) of working-class women in Camberwell. In this study, "lack of an intimate confiding relationship with a husband or boyfriend" (p. 234) was found to be one of four factors associated with increased psychiatric morbidity following stressful life events. By using this finding to support his thesis regarding the importance of attachment relationships, Henderson assumes that an intimate confiding relationship is synonymous with an attachment relationship in adults.

This general approach to attachment in adults defines attachment relationships as a subset, identified by intensity and intimacy, of an individual's social support or affiliative network. For example, in their study of "attachment and family integration," Troll and Smith (1976) accept Gewirtz's (1972) definition of attachment as a "2-person reciprocal relationship" (p. 180). The clearest statement of this understanding of attachment comes from a recent article by Heard and Lake (1986, p. 431):

> "Preferred relationships" refer to relationships in which individuals regularly expect to find opportunities for companionable and/or supportive interactions. . . . People who are so classed constitute an individual's attachment network. . . . The concept of preferred relationships in the attachment network circumvents difficulties in describing attachment relationships and affectional bonds in adults.

There are two implicit assumptions in this approach: (1) attachment can be characterized using the same criteria as affiliation (e.g., if affiliative relationships provide companionship and intimacy, attachment relationships provide preferred or more salient companionship and intimacy); and (2) attachment and affiliation serve the same function(s), with attachment again doing the job more and better (Sheldon & West, 1989). But neither of these assumptions agrees with our theoretical formulations about the nature of the attachment system in infancy and childhood.

These assumptions can lead to seemingly confusing findings in regards to the function of intimate relationships, as demonstrated by the Camberwell study of Brown and his colleagues (1975). These investigators rated "intimacy" on a 4-point scale, as Type A through Type D. Type A and Type B relationships were both defined as "close, intimate, and confiding." Type A relationships were with "husband or boyfriend, or in exceptional cases a woman with whom they lived." Type B relationships were with "mother, sister or friend whom they saw at least weekly." Only Type A relationships provide "almost complete protection" against psychiatric sequelae to stressful life events, while Type B relationships "failed to provide even relative protection" (Brown et al., 1975, p. 234).

Attachment theory can explain the difference in effectiveness between Type A and Type B relationships. In the absence of a stressor causing decreased security, Type A and Type B relationships fulfill similar affiliative needs equally well. But when a stressor activates the attachment system, attachment needs—that is, the need to reestablish a sense of security—predominate. Only Type A relationships have predominant attachment components and thus fulfill attachment needs. The findings of the Camberwell study can therefore be understood as differentiating the attachment versus affiliative components of close relationships.

As implied in the discussion of the Camberwell study, relationships can look equivalent when classified only according to affectional components but nonetheless can be quite different in terms of the ability to fulfill attachment functions. In accordance with the implications of Bowlby's theory, the principal function of adult attachment is protection from danger (as it is during childhood), although adults recognize other dangers to existence than those recognized by infants and children: specifically, threats to the individual's selfconcept and integrity (Weiss, 1982; West, Livesley, Reiffer, & Sheldon, 1986). Affiliative relationships have a quite different function, for they serve to promote exploration and expansion of interests from the secure base provided by attachment.

Theoretically, attachment in adults should be defined for investigation primarily in terms of *function* (achievement of felt security) rather than in terms of *structure* (specific behaviors or form of relationship or role-defined "other"). Any behavior be-

159

comes an attachment behavior when the purpose of the behavior is to achieve or enhance security through proximity to a particular person. Any relationship *may* have an attachment component to the degree that the relationship promotes security. A behavioral repertoire becomes an attachment pattern when it is used preferentially and consistently in an effort to achieve security (even in the face of persistent failure). A relationship becomes an attachment relationship when the primary purpose of the relationship is the provision of security.

EMPIRICAL DEMONSTRATION OF THE FUNCTIONAL DISTINCTION OF ATTACHMENT AND AFFILIATION

We conducted a study to investigate whether adults perceive functional differences between attachment and affiliative relationships. College students acted as judges to categorize 43 phrases describing characteristics of social relationships. The number of students assigning each phrase to the category associated with an attachment relationship was examined, with particular reference to those phrases ascribed by theory to attachment relationships. Our central question was: Do adults organize their expectations of relationships in a manner that reflects the functions hypothesized to characterize attachment relationships? In particular, we questioned whether these college students would distinguish function between attachment relationships and close affiliative relationships.

Forty-five terms (descriptors) used to describe the functions and characteristics of various social relationships were culled from articles in professional journals. An informal content analysis of approximately 40 articles dealing with social support, attachment, and affiliation, published over the last 2 decades in major periodicals in medicine and the social sciences (primarily psychiatry and psychology), resulted in a list of over 100 terms used to describe relationships. The review was focused particularly to find terms used to characterize the functions of social relationships for adults. From this long list of terms, a "short list" of 45 descriptors were chosen, based on relevance to functional distinctions and frequency of appearance in the literature. The intent was to be representative rather than inclusive.

The works of Bowlby, Ainsworth, and Weiss constituted the primary references for the descriptors associated theoretically with attachment relationships. These "attachment descriptors" are characteristics associated with the unique function of the attachment system (i.e., protection from dangers) and the unique goal of the attachment system (i.e., security); the attachment descriptors constituted 17 of the 45 descriptors (see Table 10.1 and Table 10.2).

One hundred fifty-three student volunteers from an undergraduate psychology course at the University of Calgary completed the simple paper-and-pencil categorization task. The students were asked to assign each term to one or more categories according to which category they felt the term would *best* apply to in their own life. The categories were "lover," "best friend," and "friend." The students were allowed to assign each descriptor to more than one category.

The instructions emphasized two points: first, that the term "lover" should be taken to signify "someone you would feel 'in love' with" rather than, necessarily, "a person you have a physical relationship with"; and second, that "we want you to decide whether *for you* in your own life the descriptor would *best* apply to someone who was your lover, best friend, or friend."

College students were well suited to function as judges for this task. The students have comparable levels of reading skills, so they could understand the task fairly easily. Most students were

TABLE 10.1. Descriptors Associated with Attachment Functions and Goal

Long-lived tie, enduring	Permanent relationship
Sexual intimacy	Provides sense of security
You fear loss of this person	Provides opportunity
Provides sense	for giving nurturance
of being needed	Separation causes distress
Caregiver	Faithful
Prevents loneliness	Sought out in times of stress
His or her happiness is	Plan future with
a goal for you	You protest separation from
You try to protect	Exclusive relationship

TABLE 10.2. Descriptors Associated with Nonattachment Functions

Important as unique individual	Loyal
Shares common interests	You cherish
Offers help when needed	Mutually confiding about personal
Competitive at times	thoughts and feelings
Loss causes grief	Frequently sought out
Frequent shared activities	Cooperative
Provides guidance and advice	Prevents isolation
Wants to maintain closeness	Provides you with a sense of worth
Independent	and competence
Companionship	Pleasure, joy in reunion
Mutual trust	Comfortable
Provides reassurance	Shared interpretation of experience
Shared activities are most important	Predictable
part of relationship	Variable and equivalent relationship
Helps you be sociable	Fixed and complementary
Knows a lot about you	relationship

18 or 24 years old; this age range is appropriate to the task because most subjects will have formed specific ideas about types of relationships, but these ideas will not ordinarily have been greatly modified by contradictory environmental responses. That is, the subjects' ideas about the functions of different types of relationship should reflect generalized expectations (i.e., working models) at least as much as practical experience.

The categories for the sorting task were chosen to represent common-language equivalents for three major types of social relationships for adults: "lover" was chosen to represent the unique pair-bonded relationship that would ordinarily constitute the attachment relationship; "best friend" was chosen to represent the close affectional and confidante relationship(s) within a social support system; "friend" was chosen to represent other, more indefinite relationships within a social support system.

The terms can be thought of as representing points on several possible continuums: least interchangeable to most interchangeable; most frequent contact to least frequent contact; most permanent to least permanent; highly physically involved to low physical involvement, and so on. So attachment functions are not necessarily a primary underlying construct in differentiating any of these types of relationships. But if attachment functions continue in adulthood, as they are in childhood, to be associated with one particular other, then the functions characteristic of attachment relationships should be associated primarily with one particular relationship, namely, the lover. This task therefore investigated the extent to which young adult judges associate attachment functions uniquely with a particular social relationship, represented by the word "lover."

Demography of the Sample

The questionnaires asked only for the age and sex of the respondents, so these are the only demographic characteristics considered. Table 10.3 relates these two demographic variables for these respondents. Females constitute 55% of the respondents; males, 37%. Twelve returns (8%) were unmarked as to age and sex.

As Table 10.3 reveals, a *t*-test indicated that age is not significantly different for females and males.

Results

Two related descriptors, Variable and Equivalent Relationship and Fixed and Complementary Relationship, were excluded from the analysis, because most subjects either ignored them or indicated confusion as to their meaning. The set of variables analyzed therefore comprised 17 variables related to functions of the attachment system and 26 variables related to functions of other social systems. Table 10.4 presents the overall percentage of subjects assigning each variable to each of the three summary categories. The variables are listed in decreasing order of assignment to the category of LOV.

TABLE 10.3. Sex and Age of Respondents

| | N | Age | | *t* value | *p* value |
		Mean	Standard deviation		
Females	84	21.7	5.9		
Males	57	20.6	3.3	1.41	0.2
Unknown	12				
Total	153	21.3	5.0		

TABLE 10.4. Percentage of All Judges Assigning Each Variable to Each Category

Variables	Categories		
	LOV	L + BF	OTH
Sexual intimacy*	97	3	0
Plan future with*	74	16	10
Exclusive relationship*	70	20	10
You protest separation from*	66	26	8
Separation causes distress*	64	29	7
His or her happiness is a goal for you*	61	30	9
Provides opportunity for giving nurturance*	55	30	15
Provides sense of being needed*	49	32	19
Provides sense of security*	44	34	22
Faithful*	43	36	20
Caregiver*	39	37	24
You cherish	37	48	15
You fear loss of this person*	33	47	20
Permanent relationship*	33	41	25
Wants to maintain closeness	33	58	10
You try to protect*	28	40	32
Frequently sought out	26	45	30
Pleasure, joy in reunion	26	47	28
Shared interpretation of experience	24	35	41
Long-lived tie, enduring*	22	45	33
Shared activities are most important part	21	27	53
Loyal	20	45	36
Prevents loneliness*	19	26	55
Sought out in times of stress*	19	47	34
Mutually confiding about personal thoughts and feelings	18	68	14
Provides you with a sense of worth and competence	18	52	30
Predictable	17	33	50
Companionship	17	30	53
Mutual trust	16	56	28
Provides reassurance	16	45	39
Frequent shared activities	14	44	42
Knows a lot about you	13	71	16
Loss causes grief	12	42	45
Cooperative	11	25	64
Important as unique individual	10	46	44
Prevents isolation	10	20	70

(cont.)

TABLE 10.4. (cont.)

	Categories		
Variables	LOV	L + BF	OTH
Independent	9	8	83
Comfortable	8	46	46
Provides guidance and advice	7	26	67
Shares common interests	5	29	66
Offers help when needed	5	39	56
Helps you be sociable	5	11	84
Competitive at times	4	9	86

Note. Variables followed by asterisks are related to attachment functions.

The first 11 variables in this ordered list are from the set of attachment variables. The last 19 variables are from the set of nonattachment variables. This simple ranking therefore presents immediate strong evidence that attachment functions are recognized implicitly by these judges as constituting a special subset of functions particularly associated with a special relationship.

Seventeen descriptors were placed in both categories of lover and best friend more often than in any other category or combination of categories. This pattern of categorization reflects the extensive functional overlap between attachment and affiliative relationships for adults in our culture. The relationship of lover is expected to fulfill the same function as the relationship of best friend. But the relationship of lover is also associated with the extra and unique functions characteristic of attachment.

Fourteen descriptors were placed in the friend category (either that category only or that category in combination with best friend, or both best friend and lover).[1] This reflects functions assigned to general social relationships. Five variables were placed in these categories by over two-thirds of the judges; these variables are: competitive at times, independent, helps you to be sociable, prevents isolation, and comfortable. The association of these functions with general social relationships has a face validity that lends credence to the general approach. The statistical significance of these results, across all ages and both genders, was confirmed using a nonparametric analysis of variance.

The results of this study can be compared with Weiss's (1982) characterization of attachment relationships for adults. Two of the characteristics that Weiss describes as common to infant and adult attachment can be related directly to terms endorsed for lover only: secure base with "provides sense of security" and separation protest with "you protest separation from" and "separation causes distress." The third characteristic that according to Weiss is shared by infant and adult attachment, proximity-seeking, does not seem to be associated exclusively with the attachment relationship by these judges, as the terms "frequently sought out," "sought out when stressed," and "wants to maintain closeness" were each endorsed for both lover and best friend.

One interpretation of these results is that close affiliative relationships include the expectation of frequent contact but not the expectation that this contact is guaranteed or will necessarily always be available when wanted or in the future. In contrast, the association of the terms "plan future with," "faithful," and "caregiver" with the lover category suggests that adults expect attachment relationships to provide availability and security not only in the present but also in the future. Expectations of a shared future appears to be a crucial hallmark of adult attachment relationships.

As we saw in Chapter 1, Weiss also identified three characteristics that differentiated adult from infant attachment: Adult attachments are typically peer relationships, involve a sexual relationship, and do not overwhelm other behaviorally based systems to the extent that infant attachment can do in times of stress. The peer relationship component is indicated in these results by the expectation of reciprocity: "his or her happiness is a goal for you," "opportunity to give nurturance," and "provides you with a sense of being needed," — all of which were preferentially endorsed for the category of lover. The term "sexual intimacy" indicates the close association of a sexual relationship with the category of lover (a finding that accentuates the obvious!); the terms "exclusive" and "faithful," endorsed preferentially for lover, can also be interpreted as relating to the sexual component of the relationship. The third characteristic identified by Weiss, the decreased ability of the attachment system to overwhelm other behaviorally based systems, is not directly tested in this study, but can be inferred from the large number of functions assigned to both lover and best friend. The adult attachment and affiliative systems are not antithetical in all functions; for adults, many functions are common to the two systems. One system would not ordinarily be capable of completely overwhelming the other, in that the shared functions, at least, should be maintained. The large number of functions endorsed for both lover and best friend is therefore in agreement with Weiss's observation.

This study demonstrated that attachment relationships serve unique functions for adults; that these functions are congruent with the functions of attachment for infants; and that the attachment relationship can be defined specifically by these unique functions (related to protection from "danger" and maintenance/ reestablishment of security).

CONCLUSIONS

We began this book with the description of reciprocal attachment for adults, focusing on its continuity with attachment in infancy, and the importance of distinguishing the unique *function* of attachment relationships. The function of attachment, the provision of safety and security, remains constant throughout the life span, although the mechanisms for achieving this function change and develop with maturation.

We have presented evidence that young adults organize their expectations of relationships in a manner congruent with a functionally distinct role for attachment. A small number of functions, of the type promoting general sociability, were common expectations of all relationships. A larger set of functions, including the provision of support and comfort, were common to only the two more personal relationships. And a specific set of functions, congruent with the theoretically defined function of attachment, were expected only of the most intimate relationship (Sheldon & West, 1989).

We have also considered the usefulness of attachment theory in differentiating personality disorders. The definition and differentiation of personality disorders remains a difficult problem in psychiatry. Vaillant and Perry (1980, p. 1563) stated that these disorders "continually demonstrate to mental health professionals the limits of their expertise, yet no group of emotional disorders is more often encountered in psychiatric practice." We have demonstrated that attachment theory contains information that is essential to understanding and classifying these disorders.

The fact that patterns of dysfunctional attachment do relate in meaningful ways to personality disorders suggests that attachment can be used both to refine diagnostic criteria and to direct treatment and intervention efforts.

For all of these purposes — attachment as a buffer for life crises, attachment as diagnostic criteria, and attachment as a therapeutic construct — the necessary prerequisite is the classification of adult attachment patterns, using techniques that are valid, reliable, and accessible to the clinician. We have presented some of our own work and the work of others in this area. But this is a relatively new and developing field in adult psychology. No book can hope to stay current — or even to be current by the time it reaches the market — on the varieties of ways of assessing adult attachment. Indeed, it was not our intention to present a comprehensive review of available instruments, but rather to focus on instruments we know to be useful in investigating the theoretical and practical aspects of attachment theory applied to adulthood.

Although, as noted by Bretherton (1992), it is conventional to date the beginning of attachment theory with *Maternal Care and Mental Health* (Bowlby, 1951), Bowlby was consistently interested since the mid-1930s in the importance of separation and loss in children's lives and their bearing on adult disorders. His early case studies as set forth in *Personality and Mental Illness* (1942) prepared the ground for the critique of the sexual etiology hypothesis of neurosis and for the accent on the effect of disruptions of the tie to parental figures in childhood and adult psychopathology. Suttie (1935) took the same position when he espoused an innate need for companionship with separation from the mother leading to long-term effects on the developing personality.

Bowlby's scientific perspective was a product of the predominant paradigms of post-World War II British science: ethology and information processing. Within the field of child psychiatry, Bowlby and his team shifted the focus from the exclusively internal to the external: Real events and relationships do play a deterministic role in development and mental health. The leading psychoanalytic theorists of the time emphasized the internal reality to the exclusion of influence from the external reality. Bowlby used ethology and evolutionary requirements as the foundation for his theory. It provided a firm foundation, but not a necessary one: Winnicott, a pediatrician turned psychoanalyst, was reaching much the same conclusions about the primacy and long-lasting effects of the infant–mother relationship without recourse to ethological theories.

To explain the varieties of expression this eminently straightforward system can take by adulthood, Bowlby turned to the other popular paradigm: information processing. As a science, information processing emerged full grown, like Athena from the head of Zeus, at the end of World War II (Campbell, 1989; Hofstadter, 1979). Bowlby used the mechanics of information processing, particularly selective exclusion of information from attention, to characterize the defensive processes that shaped the expression of attachment behaviors in adulthood.

Unfortunately, these two approaches leave "man qua man" as the missing link in the theories. The ethological approach rests on the primacy of the influence of differential contributions to survival to reproductive age. Observations from other species, particularly higher primates, were extrapolated to humans. The concepts were modified as necessary to take into account the "self-awareness" of the human, but the mechanisms were not theorized to be different because of this self-awareness: Man's behaviors were organized to promote survival of the species. This is the study of "man qua animal."

In contrast, the information-processing approach rested on the primacy of symbolic logic and algorithmic approaches to problem solving in the design of "thinking machines." The key to artificial intelligence was thought to reside in increasing the sophistication of the logic systems underlying computer programming. Similarly, the key to understanding human intelligence was thought to reside in understanding the mechanisms used by humans to make decisions. Little attention was paid to "irrelevant" accomplishments of the human intellect such as perceptions, emotions, and intuition (Campbell, 1989). This is the study of "man qua machine."

Both approaches fall short of the study of "man qua man." It is difficult to cross the boundary from nonhuman to human and still to know what and how to study humanness. It is easier — and usually more fruitful and more defensible — to study humans using the same paradigms and methods as have proven useful in the study of other phenomena, be that phenomena animal or machine. Valuable contributions can derive from such studies; but the value of the contributions is undermined when the limitations of application to humans are not understood and acknowledged.

Two examples, one from each field, can illustrate the limitations of application. From ethology we can consider the implications for man of *neoteny*. Neoteny, that is, the persistence of the characteristics of childhood (e.g., curiosity, learning) beyond the age of sexual maturity, is not found in any other species to the extent that it is found in humans (Bateson, 1979). One might expect that in humans, because of the persistence of a childlike ability to learn, the influence of the early bond may be more susceptible to modification by later experiences than is true for other species.

From the field of information processing we must take into account the recent work on the nature of intelligence and the structure of the brain (Brown & Oaksford, 1990; Campbell, 1989). This work emphasizes the inappropriateness — and lack of utility — of modeling the brain as a machine rather than as a biological product of evolutionary constraints. The way we think cannot be divorced from the physical structure of the brain or the constraints of necessary biological adaptation. But Bowlby's model of defenses as a variety of information processing is a direct progeny of attempts to model intelligence as the product of an efficient machine that functions according to general rules of logic and set algorithms. Since we now know that these concepts do not work well as models of how the brain works, we must question the utility of modeling defenses according to information-processing theory.

So we are left with two "more than" statements: Attachment for humans is more than attachment for other species and more than early infant–mother relationships. The varieties of expression of attachment for humans is more than the product of information-processing protocols of the brain.

The "bottom line," to use a modern locution, is that patterns of attachment exist and can be observed and measured. Why such patterns should exist is a matter for speculation; it does not make much difference to the existence and effects of the patterns if the answer to the question of origin is found in ethology, psychoanalytic theory, or, for that matter, religion. The *why* is a matter for philosophy; the *how* and *therefore* is a matter for developmental psychology.

EPILOGUE

I f we look for a pervasive concern or *ethic* in Bowlby's writings, we can find it in the hold that was exerted over him by the powerful way in which individual lives are shaped by the quality of parental care. This was one issue on which his scientific work gave him a right to pronounce. In *A Secure Base* (1988b, p. 2) he wrote:

> To be a successful parent means a lot of very hard work. Looking after a baby or toddler is a twenty-four hour-a-day job seven days a week, and often a very worrying one at that. Study after study . . . attest[s] that healthy, happy, and self-reliant adolescents and young adults are the products of stable homes in which both parents give a great deal of time and attention to the children.

A good deal of what has been described in the present book bears upon the effects of common variations in the way the primary caregiver responds to the child's attachment needs.

The loss of a responsive child–caregiver relationship was obvious in all the cases presented in Chapter 2. Repetitive feelings patterns such as angry yearning, guilt, fearsome possessiveness, and despair were the reaction to these losses and predominated throughout these individual's lives. Such feelings were always just around the corner awaiting expression in current relationships. A large part of the description of insecure patterns of attachment is thus an account of the repetition of feelings that create a representational identity between the individual's past and present attachment experiences.

172

Sadness, suffering, psychotherapy — all these lead us to take a second look at ourselves, to examine more carefully what we remember and feel, to understand what we have deeply longed for but missed; and all this is called mourning. The ability to experience and endure grief is the price of its relief: "He oft finds med'cine who his grief imparts" (Spencer's "The Faerie Queen," cited in Bowlby, 1980, p. 172). No less important is the presence of a trusted helping agent who is prepared to go through the process of mourning with the individual so that "the deep vase of chilling tears that grief hath shaken into frost" may break (Tennyson's "In Memoriam," cited in Bowlby, 1980, p. 320).

APPENDIX A

ITEMS ON THE RECIPROCAL ATTACHMENT QUESTIONNAIRE FOR ADULTS

DIMENSIONS OF ATTACHMENT

Proximity Seeking

> I have to have to have my attachment figure with me when I'm upset.
> I feel lost if I'm upset and my attachment figure is not around.
> When I am anxious I desperately need to be close to my attachment figure.

Separation Protest

> I don't object when my attachment figure goes away for a few days.
> I resent it when my attachment figure spends time away from me.
> I feel abandoned when my attachment figure is away for a few days.

Feared Loss

> I have a terrible fear that my relationship with my attachment figure will end.
> I'm afraid that I will lose my attachment figure's love.
> I'm confident that my attachment figure will always love me.

Availability

> I'm confident that my attachment figure will try to understand my feelings.

I worry that my attachment figure will let me down.

When I'm upset, I am confident my attachment figure will be there to listen to me.

Use

I turn to my attachment figure for many things, including comfort and reassurance.

I talk things over with my attachment figure.

Things have to be really bad for me to ask my attachment figure for help.

PATTERNS OF ATTACHMENT

Angry Withdrawal

I wish there was less anger in my relationship with my attachment figure.

I get frustrated when my attachment figure is not around as much as I would like.

My attachment figure only seems to notice me when I'm angry.

I'm furious that I don't get any comfort from my attachment figure.

I get really angry at my attachment figure because I think he or she could make more time for me.

I often feel angry with my attachment figure without knowing why.

My attachment figure is always disappointing me.

Compulsive Care Giving

I put my attachment figure's needs before my own.

I can't get on with my work if my attachment figure has a problem.

I enjoy taking care of my attachment figure.

I expect my attachment figure to take care of his or her own problems.

I don't make a fuss over my attachment figure.

I don't sacrifice my own needs for the benefit of my attachment figure.

It makes be feel important to be able to do things for my attachment figure.

Compulsive Self-Reliance

I feel it is best not to depend on my attachment figure.

I want to get close to my attachment figure, but I keep pulling back.

I wouldn't want my attachment figure relying on me.

I usually discuss my problems and concerns with my attachment figure.

It's easy for me to be affectionate with my attachment figure.

I'm so used to doing things on my own that I don't ask my attachment figure for help.

I feel that there is something wrong with me because I'm remote from my attachment figure.

Compulsive Care Seeking

I often feel too dependent on my attachment figure.

I wish that I could be a child again and be taken care of by my attachment figure.

I rely on myself and not my attachment figure to solve my problems.

I do not need my attachment figure to take care of me.

I'm never certain about what I should do until I talk to my attachment figure.

I would be helpless without my attachment figure.

I feel that the hardest thing to do is to stand on my own.

APPENDIX B

ITEMS ON THE AVOIDANT ATTACHMENT QUESTIONNAIRE FOR ADULTS

Maintains Distance in Relationships

Closeness to others frightens me because they may reject me.
I don't let anyone get close to me.
I'm afraid of getting close to others.
I have a hard time giving affection to someone.
I've built a wall around myself.
Whenever I feel myself getting close to someone, I push them away.

High Priority on Self-Sufficiency

I look to others for support.
I only feel secure when I'm by myself.
I take great pride in not needing anyone.
My strength comes only from myself.
I don't need anyone.
I get my sense of security from myself.

Attachment Relationship Is a Threat to Securtiy

Caring for someone would make me feel weak and exhausted.
Being close to someone makes me think of suffocation.
I would lose my feeling of security if I had to share my life with
    someone.
I'm afraid to care for someone because I would lose myself.
Needing someone would make me feel weak.

Desire for Close Affectional Bonds

> I wish I had someone with whom I could share my whole life.
> I wish that I had a single lasting relationship.
> It bothers me that I have no close ties to anyone.
> I long for someone to share my feelings with.
> I wish there was someone close who needed me.

APPENDIX C

NONVERBAL STIMULI
TO EVOKE INFORMATION
ON ATTACHMENT

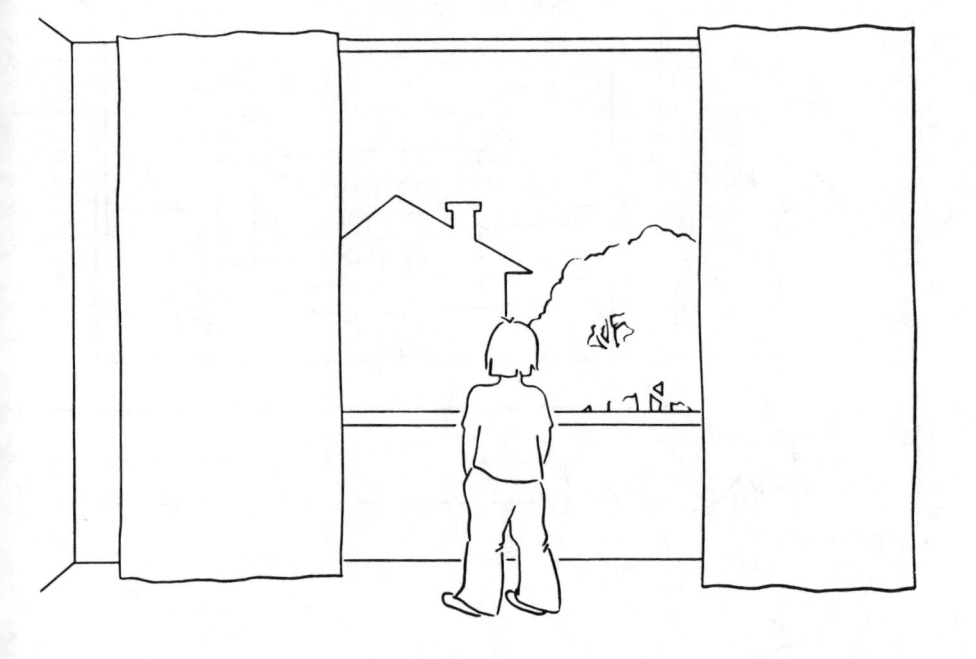

Child at window.

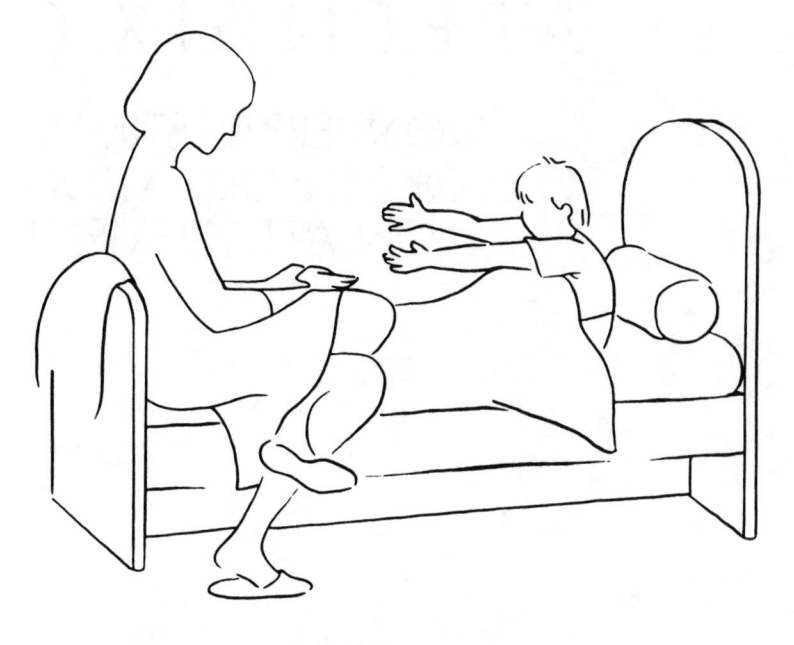

Bedtime scene.

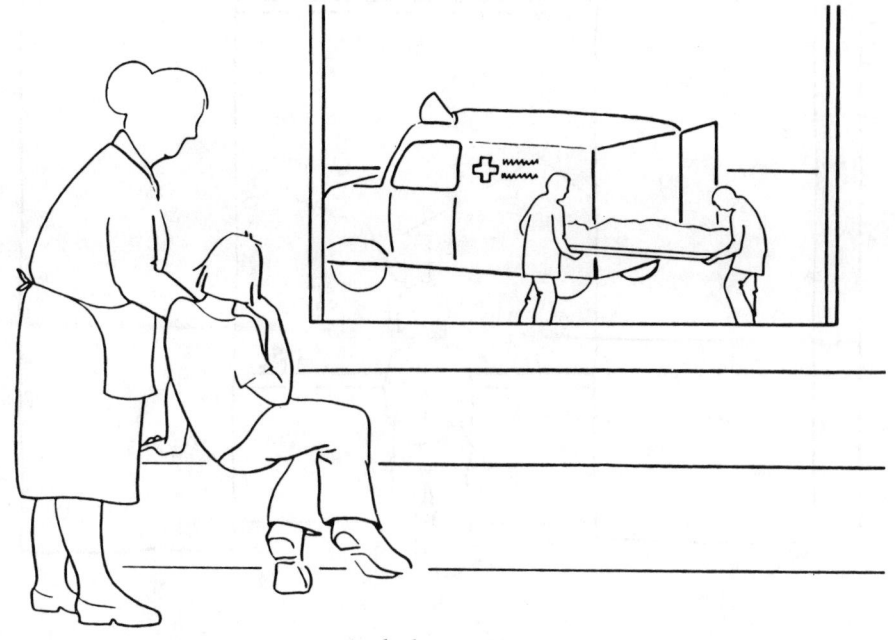

Ambulance scene.

APPENDIX D
EVALUATION OF OUTCOME

Conceptualizing the tasks of psychotherapy in attachment terms offers advantages for the evaluation of therapeutic effectiveness. The most obvious advantage is the focus provided by attachment theory: Rather than defining outcome in general terms, such as increased social network or increased self-esteem, outcome can be defined in terms of the permeability of the individual's working model of attachment. Success is operationalized as an increase in this permeability.

Theoretically, this is clear and closely related to attachment theory. But practically, a question remains: "Can the permeability be validly and reliably measured?" The empirical measures to capture working models of attachment can provide a multimethod assessment package that offers the researcher demonstrable validity and reliability. Thus, the measurement of attitudes and beliefs relevant to adult reciprocal attachment is cross-validated with the measurement of patterns of insecure attachment. Main's (1985) Adult Attachment Interview interprets the present working model based on the nature of memories of parental attachment. Therefore, the researcher interested in evaluating outcome has available several measurement tools, each with a different operational focus but each based on the same theoretical model of attachment.

NOTES

CHAPTER 1. THE DEFINITION OF ADULT RECIPROCAL ATTACHMENT

1. Throughout this book the child is referred to as masculine solely for the sake of convenience.

CHAPTER 3. DEVELOPMENTAL PERSPECTIVES

1. Relatedness in its broad outline is universally polarized in opposing tendencies, between self-definition and the desire to integrate another person into one's life. In patterns of insecure attachment, we often find the predominance of one tendency over the other, but in their varied expressions they are all-pervasive in the psychology of attachment relationships. Current psychoanalysts seem to take the same view of the matter, identifying attachment and autonomy conflicts as universal themes in every psychotherapy (Gill, 1983; Modell, 1990).

CHAPTER 4. REPRESENTATIONAL OR WORKING MODELS

1. Impressed by the metaphor of the mind as a computer, psychologists within the social cognitive frame of reference have favored an information-processing approach to interpersonal behavior. They have been most concerned with schematic processing and, in keeping with a "faulty computer" metaphor, errors in social judgment. As we have seen, this analogy is not in keeping with current models of how the brain works.

Along with this emphasis on an information-processing model of the mind, social cognitive researchers have generally applied their concepts and methods to the study of affiliative relationships. In Chapter 10 we suggest that affiliation and attachment are two different forms of relationships, best understood and investigated as distinct in function and expectations.

For both of these reasons, social cognitive research does not appear to be relevant for dealing with representations of attachment, particularly the affective component always entwined in patterns of attachment. The interested reader should consult Higgins and Bargh (1987), Markus and Zajonc (1985), and Sherman, Judd, and Park (1989) for reviews on social cognition.

2. The conception of structure, that is, the degree of differentiation in the level of representation, may be closer to the heart of the devotee of elegant theory than to the clinician faced with the practical problem of making sense of a person's attachment experiences. A concentration on the structuring of a person's working model presents us with a cross-sectional breaking out of a part from the individual's overall attachment experience. Such static understanding may not be very useful to the clinician, who is typically more concerned with genetic understanding (or helping people perceive the continuity of their attachment stories).

3. For a consideration of the meaning of this understanding of memory in the context of psychoanalytic theory, the reader is referred to Modell (1990).

CHAPTER 5. PATTERNS OF INSECURE ATTACHMENT

1. For a review of this research, see Bretherton (1985), Belsky and Nezworski (1987), Goldberg (1991), and van Ijzendoorn, Goldberg, Kroonenberg, and Frenkel (1992).

CHAPTER 9. ATTACHMENT AND PSYCHOTHERAPY

1. For the application of attachment theory to family therapy, see Heard (1982) and Byng-Hall (1991).

2. Eagle (1984) introduced the term "enactment" to refer to what we have called "modes of action" or "behavioral initiatives."

CHAPTER 10. BOUNDARIES OF ATTACHMENT

1. The combination of "lover" and "friend," without the inclusion of "best friend," did not occur for any variable.

REFERENCES

Ainsworth, M. D. S. (1968). Object relations, dependency, and attachment: A theoretical review of the infant–mother relationship. *Child Development, 40,* 969–1025.

Ainsworth, M. D. S. (1972). Attachment and dependency: A comparison. In J. L. Gewirtz (Ed.), *Attachment and dependency* (pp. 97–137). Washington, DC: Winston.

Ainsworth, M. D. S. (1985). Attachment across the life span. *Bulletin of the New York Academy of Medicine, 61,* 792–812.

Ainsworth, M. D. S. (1989). Attachments beyond infancy. *American Psychologist, 44,* 709–716.

Ainsworth, M. D. S. (1990). Epilogue. In M. T. Greenberg, D. Cicchetti, & E. M. Cummings (Eds.), *Attachment in the preschool years.* Chicago: University of Chicago Press.

Ainsworth, M. D. S., & Bell, S. M. (1970). Attachment, exploration and separation: Illustrated by the behaviour of one-year-olds in a strange situation. *Child Development, 41,* 49–67.

Ainsworth M. D. S., Blehar, M. C., Waters, E., & Wall, S. (1978). *Patterns of attachment: A psychological study of the strange situation.* Hillsdale, NJ: Erlbaum.

Ainsworth, M. D. S., & Wittig, B. A. (1969). Attachment and exploratory behaviour of one-year-olds in a strange situation. In B. M. Foss (Ed.), *Determinants of infant behaviour* (pp. 113–136). London: Methuen.

American Psychiatric Association. (1980). *Diagnostic and statistical manual of mental disorders* (3rd ed.). Washington, DC: Author.

American Psychiatric Association. (1987). *Diagnostic and statistical manual of mental disorders* (3rd ed., rev.). Washington, DC: Author.

Aquila, R. E. (1983). *Representational mind: A study of Kant's theory of knowledge.* Bloomington: Indiana University Press.

Ayer, A. J. (1946). *Language, truth and logic.* New York: Penguin Books.

Balint, M. (1968). *The basic fault: Therapeutic aspects of regression.* London: Tavistock.

Bartholomew, K. (1990). Avoidance of intimacy: An attachment perspective. *Journal of Social and Personal Relationships, 7,* 147–178.

Bartlett, F. C. (1932). *Remembering: A study in experimental and social psychology.* Cambridge, England: Cambridge University Press.

Bates, J. E., Freeland, C. A. B., & Lounsbury, M. L. (1979). Measurement of infant difficultness. *Child Development, 50,* 794–803.

Bateson, G. (1979). *Mind and nature: A necessary unity.* New York: Dutton.

Belsky, J., & Nezworski, T. (Eds.). (1987). *Clinical implications of attachment.* Hillsdale, NJ: Erlbaum.

Blanck, G., & Blanck, R. (1974). *Ego psychology: Theory and practice.* New York: Columbia University Press.

Blass, R. B., & Blatt, S. J. (1990). Attachment and separatedness: A dialectic model of the products and processes of development throughout the life cycle. *Psychoanalytic Study of the Child, 45,* 107–127.

Blatt, S. J., & Lerner, H. (1983). Investigations in the psychoanalytic theory of object relations and object representations. In J. Masling (Ed.), *Empirical studies of psychoanalytic theories* (pp. 187–249). Hillsdale, NJ: Erlbaum.

Bobrow, D. G., & Collins, A. (Eds.). (1975). *Representation and understanding: Studies in cognitive science.* New York: Academic Press.

Bowlby, J. (1942). *Personality and mental illness.* New York: Emerson Books.

Bowlby, J. (1951). *Maternal care and mental health.* Geneva, Switzerland: World Health Organization.

Bowlby, J. (1958). The nature of the child's tie to the mother. *International Journal of Psycho-Analysis, 39,* 350–369.

Bowlby, J. (1963). Pathological mourning and childhood mourning. *Journal of the American Psychoanalytic Association, 11,* 500–541.

Bowlby J. (1969/1982). *Attachment and loss: Vol. 1. Attachment.* New York: Basic Books.

Bowlby J. (1973). *Attachment and loss: Vol. 2. Separation: Anxiety and anger.* New York: Basic Books.

Bowlby, J. (1977). The making and breaking of affectional bonds. *British Journal of Psychiatry, 130,* 201–210, 421–431.

Bowlby, J. (1979a). By ethology out of psychoanalysis: An experiment in interbreeding. *Animal Behavior, 28,* 649–656.

Bowlby, J. (1979a). By ethology out of psychoanalysis: An experiment in interbreeding. *Animal Behavior, 28,* 649–656.

Bowlby J. (1980). *Attachment and loss: Vol. 3. Loss, sadness and depression.* New York: Basic Books.

Bowlby J. (1988a). Developmental psychiatry comes of age. *American Journal of Psychiatry, 145,* 1–10.

Bowlby, J. (1988b). *A secure base.* New York: Basic Books.

Braito, R., Breci, M., & Keith, P. M. (1990). Rethinking isolation among the married and the unmarried. *American Journal of Orthopsychiatry, 60,* 289–297.

Brenner, C. (1955). *An elementary textbook of psychoanalysis.* New York: International Universities Press.

Bretherton. I. (1985). Attachment theory: Retrospect and prospect. In I. Bretherton & E. Waters (Eds.), *Growing points of attachment theory and research. Monographs of the Society for Research in Child Development, 50* (1–2, Serial No. 209), 3–35.

Bretherton, I. (1992). The origins of attachment theory: John Bowlby and Mary Ainsworth. *Developmental Psychology, 28,* 759–775.

Brown G. W., Bhrolchain, M. N., & Harris, T. (1975). Social class and psychiatric disturbance among women in an urban population. *Sociology, 9,* 225–254.

Brown, G. D. A., & Oaksford, M. (1990). Representational systems and symbolic systems. *Behavior and Brain, 13,* 492.

Byng-Hall, J. (1991). The application of attachment theory to understanding and treatment in family therapy. In C. M. Parkes, J. Stevenson-Hinde, & P. Marris (Eds.), *Attachment across the life cycle* (pp. 199–215). New York: Routledge.

Cairns, R. (1972). Attachment and dependency: A psychobiological and social-learning synthesis. In J. Gewirtz (Ed.), *Attachment and dependency* (pp. 29–80). Washington, DC: Winston.

Campbell, J. (1989). *The improbable machine.* New York: Simon & Schuster.

Caplan, G. (1974). *Support systems and community mental health.* New York: Behavioral Publications.

Cassidy, J., & Kobak, R. (1987). Avoidance and its relation to other defensive processes. In J. Belsky & T. Nezworski (Eds.), *Clinical implications of attachment* (pp. 300–325). Hillsdale, NJ: Erlbaum.

Cohen, S., & Syme, N. (Eds.). (1985). *Social support and health.* Orlando, FL: Academic Press.

Cohn, D. (1990). Child–mother attachment of 6-year-olds and social competence at school. *Child Development, 61,* 152–162.

Craik, K. (1943). *The nature of explanation*. Cambridge, England: Cambridge University Press.

Cramer, D. (1990). Psychological adjustment, close relationships and personality. *British Journal of Medical Psychology, 63*, 341–343.

Crowell, J. A., & Feldman, S. S. (1988). Mothers' internal models of relationships and children's behavioral and developmental status: A study of mother–child interaction. *Child Development, 59*, 1273–1285.

Dahl, A. A. (1990). Empirical evidence for a core borderline syndrome. *Journal of Personality Disorders, 4*, 192–202.

Derogatis, L. R. (1977). *The SCL-90-R administration, scoring, and procedures manual*. Baltimore: Clinical Psychometric Research.

Dozier, M. (1990). Attachment organization and treatment use for adults with serious psychopathological disorders. *Development and Psychopathology, 2*, 47–60.

Draper, P., & Belsky, J. (1990). Personality development in evolutionary perspective. *Journal of Personality, 58*, 141–161.

Eagle, M. (1984). *Recent developments in psychoanalysis*. New York: McGraw-Hill.

Edelman, G. (1987). *Neural darwinism*. New York: Basic Books.

Eichenbaum, L., & Orbach, S. (1985). *Understanding women*. Harmondsworth, England: Penguin.

Endler, N. S., & Edwards, J. M. (1988). Personality disorders from an interactional perspective. *Journal of Personality Disorders, 2*, 326–333.

Engel, G. L. (1971). Attachment behavior, object relations and the dynamic-economic points of view: Critical review of Bowlby's attachment and loss. *International Journal of Psycho-Analysis, 52*, 183–196.

Erikson, M., Sroufe, A., & Egeland, B. (1986). The relationship between quality of attachment and behavior problems in preschool in a high risk sample. In I. Bretherton & E. Waters (Eds.), *Growing points in attachment theory and research. Monographs of the Society for Research in Child Development, 50* (1–2, Serial No. 209), 147–168.

Fagot, B. I., & Kavanagh, K. (1990) The prediction of antisocial behavior from avoidant attachment classifications. *Child Development, 61*, 864–883.

Fairbairn, W. (1952). *An object-relations theory of the personality*. New York: Basic Books.

Feldman, D. C., & Ingham, M. E. (1975). Attachment behavior: A validation study in two age groups. *Child Development, 45*, 319–330.

Fenichel, O. (1945). *The psychoanalytic theory of neurosis.* New York: W. W. Norton.

Frances, A. J., & Widiger, T. (1989). The classification of personality disorders: An overview of problems and solutions. *Annual Review, 5,* 241–257.

Freeman, S. J. J., & Sheldon A. E. R. (1985). Social support as a modifier of stress. *Proceedings of symposium: Current issues in occupational stress.* Toronto: York University Press.

Freud, A. (1960). Discussion of Dr. Bowlby's paper: Grief and mourning in infancy and early childhood. *Psychoanalytic Study of the Child, 15,* 53–62.

Freud, A., & Dann, S. (1951). An experiment in group upbringing. *Psychoanalytic Study of the Child, 6,* 127–168.

Freud, S. (1926). Inhibitions, symptoms and anxiety. In J. Strachey (Ed. and Trans.), *The standard edition of the complete psychological works of Sigmund Freud* (Vol. 20, pp. 77–175). London: Hogarth Press, 1959.

Freud, S. (1933). New introductory lectures on psycho-analysis. In J. Strachey (Ed. and Trans.), *The standard edition of the complete psychological works of Sigmund Freud* (Vol. 22, pp. 1–182). London: Hogarth Press, 1964.

Freud, S. (1940). An outline of psycho-analysis. In J. Strachey (Ed. and Trans.), *The standard edition of the complete psychological works of Sigmund Freud* (Vol. 23, pp. 139–207). London: Hogarth Press, 1964.

George, C., Kaplan, N., & Main, M. (1985). *Adult attachment interview.* Unpublished manuscript, Department of Psychology, University of California at Berkeley.

Gewirtz, J. L. (1972) *Attachment and dependency.* Washington, DC: Winston.

Gill, M. (1983). The point of view of psychoanalysis: Energy discharge or person. *Psychoanalysis and Contemporary Thought, 6,* 523–551.

Goldberg, S. (1991). Recent developments in attachment theory. *Canadian Journal of Psychiatry, 36,* 393–400.

Gorton, G., & Akhtar, S. (1990). The literature on personality disorders, 1985–88: Trends, issues, and controversies. *Hospital and Community Psychiatry, 41,* 39–50.

Green, J. (1986). *On private madness.* Madison, CT: International Universities Press.

Greenacre, P. (1954). The role of transference: Practical considerations in relation to psychoanalytic therapy. *Journal of the American Psychoanalytic Association, 2,* 671–684.

Greenberg, M. T., Cicchetti, D., & Cummings, E. M. (1990). *Attachment in the preschool years*. Chicago: University of Chicago Press.

Grice, H. P. (1975). *Logic and conversation*. In P. Cole & J. L. Moran (Eds.), *Syntax and semantics III: Speech acts* (pp. 41–58). New York: Academic Press.

Grossmann, K., Fremmer-Bombik, E., Rudolph, J., & Grossmann, K. E. (1988). Maternal attachment representations as related to patterns of infant–mother attachment and maternal care during the first year. In R. A. Hinde & J. Stevenson-Hinde (Eds.), *Relationships within families* (pp. 241–260). Oxford: Oxford University Press.

Guidano, V. F., & Liotti, G. (1983). *Cognitive processes and emotional disorders*. New York: Guilford Press.

Guntrip, H. (1969). *Schizoid phenomena, object-relations and the self*. New York: International Universities Press.

Guntrip, H. (1974). Psychoanalytic object relations theory: The Fairbairn-Guntrip approach. In S. Arieti (Ed.), *American handbook of psychiatry* (Vol. 1, pp. 828–842). New York: Basic Books.

Hamilton, V. (1985). John Bowlby: An ethological basis for psychoanalysis. In J. Reppen (Ed.), *Beyond Freud: A study of modern psychoanalytic theorists* (pp. 1–28). Hillsdale, NJ: Erlbaum.

Hansburg, H. G. (1972). *Adolescent separation anxiety: A method for the study of adolescent separation problems*. Springfield, IL: C. C. Thomas.

Harter, S. (1983). The development of the self-system. In M. Hetherington (Ed.), *Handbook of child psychology: Vol. 4. Social and personality development* (pp. 275–386). New York: Wiley.

Harter, S. (1986). Cognitive-developmental processes in the integration of concepts about emotions and the self. *Social Cognition, 4*, 119–151.

Hazan, C., & Shaver, P. (1987). Romantic love conceptualized as an attachment process. *Journal of Personality and Social Psychology, 52*, 511–524.

Hazan, C., & Shaver, P. R. (1990). Love and work: An attachment-theoretical perspective. *Journal of Personality and Social Psychology, 59*, 270–280.

Head, H. (1926). *Aphasia and kindred disorders of speech*. Cambridge, England: Cambridge University Press.

Heard, D. H. (1982). Family systems and the attachment dynamics. *Journal of Family Therapy, 4*, 99–116.

Heard, D. H., & Lake, B. (1986). The attachment dynamic in adult life. *British Journal of Psychiatry, 149*, 430–438.

Heil, J. (1983). *Perception and cognition.* Berkeley: University of California Press.

Henderson, S. (1977). The social network, support and neurosis: The function of attachment in adult life. *British Journal of Psychiatry, 131,* 185–191.

Henderson, S., Duncan-Jones, P., & Byrne, D. (1980). Measuring social relationships: The interview schedule for social interaction. *Psychological Medicine, 10,* 723–734.

Higgins, E. T., & Bargh, J. A. (1987). Social cognition and social perceptions. *Annual Review of Psychology, 38,* 364–426.

Hinde, R. A. (1975). The concept of function. In G. P. Baerends, C. Beer, & A. Manning (Eds.), *Function and Evolution in Behavior* (pp. 3–15). Oxford: Clarendon Press.

Hinde, R. A. (1976). On describing relationships. *Journal of Child Psychology and Psychiatry, 17,* 1–19.

Hinde, R. A. (1982). Attachment: Some conceptual and biological isues. In C. M. Parkes & J. Stevenson-Hinde (Eds.), *The place of attachment in human behavior* (pp. 60–76). New York: Basic Books.

Hinde R. A., & Stevenson-Hinde J. (1976). Towards understanding relationships: Dynamic stability. In P. P. G. Bateson & R. A. Hinde (Eds.), *Growing points in ethology* (pp. 451–479). Cambridge, England: Cambridge University Press.

Hirschfeld, R. M. A., Klerman, G. L., Gough, H. G., Barrett, J., Korchin, S. J., & Chodoff, P. (1977). A measure of interpersonal dependency. *Journal of Personality Assessment, 41,* 610–618.

Hirschfeld, R. M. A., Shea, M. T., & Weise, R. (1991). Dependent personality disorder: Perspectives for DSM-IV. *Journal of Personality Disorders, 5,* 135–149.

Hofstadter, D. (1979). *Godel, Escher, Bach: An eternal golden braid.* New York: Vintage Books.

Horowitz, M. J. (1987) *States of mind: Configurational analysis of individual psychology* (2nd ed.). New York: Plenum Press.

Horowitz, M. J. (1988). *Introduction to psychodynamics: A synthesis.* New York: Basic Books.

Jackson, D. N. (1971). The dynamics of structured tests. *Psychological Review, 78,* 229–248.

Jones, B. A. (1983). Healing factors of psychiatry in light of attachment theory. *American Journal of Psychotherapy, 37,* 235–244.

Kant, I. (1781). *Critique of pure reason.* (N. K. Smith, Trans.). New York: St. Martins Press, 1969.

Karen, R. (1990, February). Becoming attached. *Atlantic Monthly,* 35–70.

Kempson, R. M. (Ed.). (1988). *Mental representations: The interface between language and reality.* Cambridge, MA: Cambridge University Press.

Kernberg, O. (1980). *Internal world and external reality.* New York: Jason Aronson.

Khan, M. (1963). The concept of cumulative trauma. *Psychoanalytic Study of the Child, 18,* 286–306.

Klein, G. S. (1958). Cognitive control and motivation. In G. Lindzey (Ed.), *Assessment of human motives* (pp. 87–118). New York: Grove Press.

Klopfer, B., Kelley, D. M., & Davidson, H. H. (1942). *The Rorschach technique: A manual for a projective method of personality diagnosis.* Yonkers-on-Hudson, NY: World Book.

Kobak, R. R., & Sceery, A. (1988). The transition to college: Working models of attachment, affect regulation, and perceptions of self and others. *Child Development, 59,* 135–146.

Koestler, A. (1966). *The act of creation.* London: Hutchinson.

Koestler, A. (1967). *The ghost in the machine.* London: Hutchinson.

Kohut, H. (1971). *The analysis of the self.* Madison, CT: International Universities Press.

Kohut, H. (1984). *How does analysis cure?* Chicago: University of Chicago Press.

Kretschmer, E. (1925). *Physique and character: An investigation of the nature of constitution and of the theory of temperament* (2nd rev. ed.) (W. J. H. Sprott, Trans.). New York: Harcourt, Brace.

Kris, E. (1956). The recovery of childhood memories in psychoanaysis. *Psychoanalytic Study of the Child, 11,* 54–88.

Kuhn T. S. (1970). *The structure of scientific revolutions* (2nd ed.). Chicago: Chicago University Press.

Lamb, M. E. (1985). *Infant–mother attachment: The origins and developmental significance of individual differences in strange situation behavior.* Hillsdale, NJ: Erlbaum.

Lewis, M., Feiring, C., McGuffog, C., & Jaskir, J. (1984). Predicting psychopathology in six-year-olds from early social relations. *Child Development, 55,* 123–136.

Links, P. (1990). Interpersonal disorder in borderline patients. In P. Links (Ed.), *Borderline personality disorder* (pp. 27–39). Washington DC: American Psychiatric Press.

Livesley, W. J. (1987). A systematic approach to the delineation of personality disorders. *American Journal of Psychiatry, 144,* 772–777.

Livesly, W. J., & Jackson, D. N. (1992). Guidelines for developing and evaluating the classification of personality disorders. *Journal of Nervous and Mental Disease, 180,* 609–618.

Livesley W. J., Jackson D. N., & Schroeder M. L. (1989). A study of the factorial structure of personality pathology. *Journal of Personality Disorders, 3-4,* 292–306.

Livesley, W. J., Jackson, D. N., & Schroeder, M. L. (1991). Dimensions of personality pathology. *Canadian Journal of Psychiatry, 36,* 557–562.

Livesley, W. J., & Schroeder, M. L. (1991). Dimensions of personality disorders: DSM-III-R cluster B diagnoses. *Journal of Nervous and Mental Disease, 179,* 320–328.

Livesley, W. J., Schroeder, M. L. & Jackson, D. N. (1990). Dependent personality disorder and attachment problems. *Journal of Personality Disorders, 4,* 131–140.

Livesley, W. J., & West, M. L. (1987). The DSM-III distinction between schizoid and avoidant personality disorders reconsidered: A case presentation. *American Journal of Psychotherapy, 39,* 59–62.

Loevinger, J. (1957). Objective tests as instruments of psychological theory. *Psychological Reports, 78,* 635–694.

Loevinger, J. (1966). The meaning and measurement of ego development. *American Psychologist, 21,* 195–206.

Lorenz, K. (1952). *King Solomon's ring.* New York: T. Y. Crowell.

Mahler, M., Pine, F., & Bergman, A. (1975). *The psychological birth of the human infant: Symbiosis and individuation.* New York: Basic Books.

Main, M. (1977). Analysis of a peculiar form of reunion behavior in some day-care children: Its history and sequelae in children who are home-reared. In R. Webb (Ed.), *Social development in childhood: Day care programs and research* (pp. 33–78). Baltimore: Johns Hopkins University Press.

Main, M. (1981). Avoidance in the service of attachment: A working paper. In K. Immelmann, G. Barlow, L. Petrinovich, & M. Main (Eds.), *Behavioral development: The Bielefeld interdisciplinary program* (pp. 651–693). Cambridge, England: Cambridge University Press.

Main, M. (1985, April). *An adult attachment classification system: Its relation to infant–parent attachment.* Paper presented at the Biennial Meeting of the Society for Research in Child Development, Toronto, Canada.

Main, M. (1991). Metacognitive knowledge, metacognitive monitoring, and singular (coherent) vs. multiple (incoherent) models of attachment: Findings and directions for future research. In C. M. Parkes, P. Marris, & J. Stevenson-Hinde (Eds.), *Attachment across the life cycle* (pp. 127–159). New York: Routledge.

Main, M., & Cassidy, J. (1988). Categories of response to reunion with the parent at age six: Predictable from infant attachment classification and stable over a one-month period. *Developmental Psychology, 24,* 415–426.

Main, M., & Goldwyn, R. (1984). Predicting rejection of her infant from mother's representation of her own experience: Implications for the abused-abusing intergenerational cycle. *Child Abuse and Neglect, 8,* 203–217.

Main, M., & Hesse, E. (1990). Parents' unresolved traumatic experiences are related to infant disorganized attachment status: Is frightening and/or frightened parental behaviour the linking mechanism? In M. Greenberg, D. Cicchetti, & M. Cummings (Eds.), *Attachment in the preschool years* (pp. 161–182). Chicago: University of Chicago Press.

Main, M., Kaplan, N., & Cassidy, J. (1985). Security in infancy, childhood and adulthood: A move to the level of representation. In I. Bretherton & E. Waters (Eds.), *Growing points in attachment theory and research: Monographs of the Society for Social Research in Child Development, 50* (1–2, Serial No. 209), 66–104.

Main, M., & Solomon, J. (1986). Discovery of an insecure-disorganized/disoriented attachment pattern. In T. B. Brazelton & M. W. Yogman (Eds.), *Affective development in infancy* (pp. 95–124). Norwood, NJ: ABLEX.

Malan, D. (1979). *Individual psychotherapy and the science of psychodynamics.* London: Butterworths.

Markus, H., & Zajonc, R. (1985). The cognitive perspective in social psychology. In G. Lindzey & E. Aronson (Eds.), *Handbook of social psychology* (3rd ed., pp. 137–230). New York: Random House.

Masters, J., & Wellman, H. (1974). Human infant attachment: A procedural critique. *Psychological Bulletin, 81,* 218–237.

Matas, L., Arend, R., & Sroufe, L. A. (1978). Continuity of adaptation in the second year: The relationship between quality of attachment and later competent functioning. *Child Development, 49,* 547–556.

Mehrabian, A., & Karonzby, D. (1974). *A theory of affiliation.* Lexington, MA: D. C. Heath.

Melges, F., & Swartz, M. (1989). Oscillations of attachment in borderline personality disorder. *American Journal of Psychiatry, 146,* 1116–1120.

Millon, T. (1983). *Millon clinical multiaxial inventory manual* (3rd ed.). Minneapolis, MN: National Computer Systems.

Millon, T. (1987). Concluding commentary. *Journal of Personality Disorders, 1,* 110–112.

Mitchell, S. (1988). *Relational concepts in psychoanalysis: An integration.* Cambridge, MA: Harvard University Press.

Modell, A. (1976). "The holding environment" and the therapeutic action of psychoanalysis. *Journal of the American Psychoanalytic Association, 56,* 57–68.

Modell, A. (1984). *Psychoanalysis in a new context.* New York: International Universities Press.

Modell, A. (1990). *Other times, other realities.* Cambridge, MA: Harvard University Press.

Mueller, D. P. (1980). Social networks: A promising direction for research on the relationship of the social environment to psychiatric disorder. *Social Science and Medicine, 14A,* 147–161.

Murray-Parkes, C., Stevenson-Hinde, J., & Marris, P. (Eds.). (1991). *Attachment across the life cycle.* New York: Routledge.

Neisser, U. (1976). *Cognition and reality.* New York: W. H. Freeman.

Parens, H., & Saul, L. (1971). *Dependence in man.* New York: Internaional University Press.

Parkes, C. (1973). Factors determining the persistence of phantom pain in the amputee. *Journal of Psychosomatic Research, 17,* 97–108.

Perlman, D. (1988). Loneliness: A life span, family perspective. In R. M. Milardo (Ed.), *Families and social networks* (pp. 190–220). Newbury Park, CA: Sage.

Perry, J. C. (1992). Problems and considerations in the valid assessment of personality disorders. *American Journal of Psychiatry, 149,* 1645–1653.

Peterfreund, E. (1971). *Information systems and psychoanalysis. (Psychological Issues,* Vol. 7, Monogr. 25/26). New York: International Universities Press.

Peterfreund, E. (1983). *The process of psychoanalytic therapy: Models and strategies.* Hillsdale, NJ: Erlbaum.

Piaget, J. (1954). *The construction of reality in the child.* New York: Basic Books.

Pilkonis, P., & Frank, E. (1988). Personality pathology in recurrent depression: Nature, prevalence and relationship to treatment response. *American Journal of Psychiatry, 145,* 435–441.

Rapaport, D. (1959). The structure of psychoanalytic theory: A systematizing attempt. In S. Koch (Ed.), *Psychology; A study of a science* (Vol. 3, pp. 55–183). New York: McGraw-Hill.

Rice, K. G., Fitzgerald, D. P., & Lapsley, D. K. (1990). Adolescents' attachment, identity and adjustment to college: Implications for the continuity of adaptation hypothesis. *Journal of Counselling and Development, 68,* 561–565.

Ricks, M. (1985). The social transmission of parental behavior: Attachment across generations. In I. Bretherton & E. Waters (Eds.), *Growing points in attachment theory and research. Monographs of the Society for Research in Child Development, 50* (1–2, Serial No. 209), 211–227.

Rosenfield, I. (1992). *The strange, familiar and forgotten.* New York: Knopf.

Rosenstein, D., Horowitz, H. A., Steidl, J. H., & Oreston, W. F. (1992). Attachment and internalization: Relationship as a regulatory context. In S. C. Feinstein, A. H. Esman, H. A. Horowitz, J. G. Looney, G. H. Orvin, J. L. Schimel, A. Z. Schwartzberg, A. D. Sorosky, & M. Sugar (Eds.), *Adolescent psychiatry: Developmental and clinical studies* (Vol. 18, pp. 491–501). Chicago: University of Chicago Press.

Rosenthal, M. (1973). Attachment and mother–infant interaction: Some research impasses and a suggested change in orientation. *Journal of Child Psychology and Psychiatry and Allied Disciplines, 14,* 201–207.

Rumelhart, D. E. (1980). Schemata: The building blocks of cognition. In R. J. Spiro, B. Bertram, & W. F. Brewer (Eds.), *Theoretical issues in reading comprehension* (pp. 33–58). Hillsdale, NJ: Erlbaum.

Rutter, M. (1981). Attachment and the development of social relationships. In M. Rutter (Ed.), *Scientific foundations of developmental psychiatry* (pp. 267–279). Baltimore: University Park Press.

Sandler, J. (1960). The background of safety. *International Journal of Psycho-Analysis, 41,* 352–356.

Sandler, J., & Rosenblatt, B. (1962). The concept of the representational world. *Psychoanalytic Study of the Child, 17,* 128–145.

Sarason, I., & Sarason, B. (Eds.). (1985). *Social support: Theory, research and application.* The Hague, The Netherlands: Martinus Nijhoff.

Sayers, D. (1987). *The mind of the maker.* San Francisco: Harper & Row.

Schafer, R. (1983). *The analytic attitude.* New York: Basic Books.

Schiffer, S., & Steele, S. (Eds.). (1988). *Cognition and representation.* Boulder, CO: Westview Press.

Scott, J. (1988). Social network analysis. *Sociology, 22,* 109–127.

Sheldon, A. E. R., & West, M. (1988). Avoidant, schizoid and dependent personality disorders. *American Journal of Psychiatry, 145,* 276–277.

Sheldon, A. E. R., & West, M. (1989). The functional discrimination of attachment and affiliation: Theory and empirical demonstration. *British Journal of Psychiatry, 155,* 18–23.

Sheldon, A. E. R., & West, M. (1990). Attachment pathology vs. low social skills in avoidant personality disorder. *Canadian Journal of Psychiatry, 35,* 596–599.

Sherman, S. J., Judd, C. M., & Park, B. (1989). Social cognition. *Annual Review of Psychology, 40,* 281–326.

Shneidman, E. S. (Ed.) (1951). *Thematic test analysis.* New York: Grune & Stratton.

Slap, J. W., & Saykin, A. (1983). The schema: Basic concept in a non-metapsychological model of the mind. *Psychoanalysis and Contemporary Thought, 6,* 305–325.

Spence, D. (1982). *Narrative truth and historical truth.* New York: Basic Books.

Sperling, M. B., Sharp, J. L., & Fishler, P. H. (1991). On the nature of attachment in a borderline population: A preliminary report. *Psychological Reports, 68,* 543–546.

Sroufe, L. A. (1986). Bowlby's contribution to psychoanalytic theory and developmental psychopathology. *Journal of Child Psychology and Psychiatry, 27,* 841–849.

Sroufe, L. A., & Fleeson, J. (1988). The coherence of family relationships. In R. A. Hinde & J. Stevenson-Hinde (Eds.), *Relationships within families* (pp. 27–47). Oxford: Clarendon Press.

Sroufe L. A., & Waters, E. (1977). Attachment as an organizing construct. *Child Development, 48,* 1184–1199.

Stern, D. (1985). *The interpersonal world of the infant.* New York: Basic Books.

Stevenson-Hinde, J., & Hinde, R. (1990). Attachment: Biological, cultural and individual desiderata. *Human Development, 33,* 62–72.

Stewart, M. J. (1989). Social support: Diverse theoretical perspectives. *Social Science and Medicine, 28,* 1217–1282.

Stiver, I. P. (1990). *Dysfunctional families and wounded relationships.* Wellesley, MA: Stone Center Working Papers Series.

Sullivan, H. S. (1953). *The interpersonal theory of psychiatry.* New York: Norton.

Suttie, I. (1935). *The origins of love and hate.* London: Kegan, Paul, Trench, Trubner.

Tinbergen, N. (1951). *The study of instinct.* London: Oxford University Press.

Tizard, B., & Hodges, J. (1978). The effect of institutional rearing on the development of 8-year-old children. *Journal of Child Psychology and Psychiatry, 19,* 99–118.

Tomkins, S. (1961). *Affect, imagery, consciousness.* New York: Springer.

Troll, L. E., & Smith, J. (1976). Attachment through the life span: Some questions about dyadic bonds among adults. *Human Development, 19,* 156–170.

Tronick, E., & Adamson, L. (1980). *Babies as people.* New York: Collier.

Tulving, E. (1972). Episodic and semantic memory. In E. Tulving & W. Donaldson (Eds.), *Organization of memory* (pp. 382–403). New York: Academic Press.

Vaillant, G. E., & Perry, J. C. (1980). Personality disorders. In H. I. Kaplan, A. M. Freedman, & B. J. Sadock (Eds.), *Comprehensive textbook of psychiatry: Part 3, Vol. 2* (3rd ed., pp. 1562–1590). Baltimore: Williams & Wilkins.

van Ijzenoorn, M. H., Goldberg, S., Kroonenberg, P. M., & Frenkel, O. J. (1992). The relative effects of maternal and child problems on the quality of attachment: A metanalysis of attachment in clinical samples. *Child Development, 63,* 840–858.

Vaux, A. (1988). *Social support: Theory, research and intervention.* New York: Praeger.

Waddington, C. H. (1957). *The strategy of genes.* London: George Allen & Unwin.

Waddington, C. H. (1967). *Principles of development and differentiation.* New York: Macmillan.

Waters, E., & Deane, K. E. (1985). Defining and assessing individual differences in attachment relationships: Q-methods and the organization of behavior in infancy and early childhood. In I. Bretherton & E. Waters (Eds.) *Growing points in attachment theory and research. Monographs of the Society for Research in Child Development, 50* (1–2, Serial No. 209), 211–227.

Watkins, K. P. (1987). *Parent–child attachment: A guide to research.* New York: Garland.

Webb, L. J., DiClemente, C. C., Johnstone, E. E., Sanders, J. L., & Perley, R. A. (1981). *DSM-III training guide.* New York: Brunner/Mazel.

Webster's encyclopedic dictionary of the English language. (1988). Canadian ed. New York: Lexicon Publications.

Weiss, R. S. (1974). The provisions of social relationships. In Z. Rubin (Ed.), *Doing unto others* (pp. 17–26). Englewood Cliffs, NJ: Prentice-Hall.

Weiss, R. S. (1982). Attachment in adult life. In C. M. Parkes & J. Stevenson-Hinde (Eds.), *The place of attachment in human behavior* (pp. 171–184). New York: Basic Books.

Weiss, R. S. (1991). The attachment bond in childhood and adulthood. In C. M. Parkes, P. Marris, & J. Stevenson-Hinde (Eds.), *Attachment across the life cycle* (pp. 66–76). New York: Routledge.

Weiss, J., & Sampson, H. (1986) *The psychoanalytic process.* New York: Guilford Press.

Werner, H. (1948). *Comparative psychology of mental development.* Chicago: Follett.

West, M. L., & Keller, A. E. R. (1991). Parentification of the child: A case study of Bowlby's compulsive caregiving attachment pattern. *American Journal of Psychotherapy, 45,* 425–431.

West, M., Keller, A., Links, P., & Patrick, J. (1993). Borderline disorder and attachment pathology. *Canadian Journal of Psychiatry, 18,* 16–22.

West, M., Livesley, J., Reiffer, L., & Sheldon, A. E. R. (1986). The place of attachment in the life events model of stress and illness. *Canadian Journal of Psychiatry, 31,* 202–207.

West, M., & Sheldon, A. E. R. (1988). The classification of pathological attachment patterns in adults. *Journal of Personality Disorders, 2,* 153–160.

West, M., Sheldon, A. E. R., & Reiffer, L. (1987). An approach to the delineation of adult attachment: Scale development and reliability. *Journal of Nervous and Mental Disease, 175,* 738–741.

West, M., Sheldon, A. E. R., & Reiffer, L. (1989). Attachment theory and brief psychotherapy: Applying current research to clinical interventions. *Canadian Journal of Psychiatry, 34,* 369–375.

West, M., & Sheldon-Keller, A. E. R. (1992). The assessment of dimensions relevant to adult reciprocal attachment. *Canadian Journal of Psychiatry, 37,* 600–606.

Westen, D. (1990). Toward a revised theory of borderline object relations: Implications of empirical research. *International Journal of Psycho-Analysis, 71,* 661–693.

Widiger, T. A. (1992). Categorical versus dimensional classification: Implications from and for research. *Journal of Personality Disorders, 6,* 287–300.

Widiger, T. A., & Frances, A. (1985). The DSM-III personality disorders: Perspectives from psychology. *Archives of General Psychiatry, 42,* 615–623.

Widiger, T. A., & Frances, A. (1987). Interviews and inventories for the measurement of personality disorders. *Clinical Psychology Review, 1,* 49–75.

Winnicott, D. W. (1965). *The maturational process and the facilitating environment.* New York: International Universities Press.

Winnicott, D. (1986). *Holding and interpretation*. New York: Grove Press.
Young, J. Z. (1964). *A model of the brain*. Oxford: Clarendon Press.

INDEX